ALZHEIMER'S DISEASE

ALZHEIMER'S DISEASE

A Guide to Diagnosis, Treatment, and Management

James E. Soukup

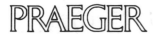

Westport, Connecticut
London

Library of Congress Cataloging-in-Publication Data

Soukup, James E.
    Alzheimer's disease : a guide to diagnosis, treatment, and
management / James E. Soukup.
        p.   cm.
    Includes bibliographical references and index.
    ISBN 0–275–95460–9 (alk. paper)
    1. Alzheimer's disease.   I. Title.
    [DNLM: 1. Alzheimer's Disease—diagnosis.   2. Alzheimer's Disease—
therapy.   WT 155 S721a 1996]
    RC523.S67   1996
    616.8'31—dc20
    DNLM/DLC
    for Library of Congress   95–49687

British Library Cataloguing in Publication Data is available.

Library of Congress Catalog Card Number: 95–49687
ISBN: 0–275–95460–9

First published in 1996

Praeger Publishers, 88 Post Road West, Westport, CT 06881
An imprint of Greenwood Publishing Group, Inc.

Printed in the United States of America

The paper used in this book complies with the
Permanent Paper Standard issued by the National
Information Standards Organization (Z39.48–1984).

10   9   8   7   6   5   4   3   2   1

*This book is dedicated to my mother,
who died of Alzheimer's disease, and
my father, who cared for her with
love and compassion for the last
seven years of her life.*

» «
====

Contents

» «

Preface

Alzheimer's disease is a progressive physical disorder which causes increasingly severe impairment in cognitive and functional ability in individuals suffering from the disorder. The onset of the disease is insidious; the course over the years is devastating. It is estimated that 4 million Americans suffer from Alzheimer's disease. The annual economic costs of care run $40 billion. The emotional cost to family and the individuals suffering from the disorder is beyond estimation.

However, Alzheimer's disease is often misdiagnosed. An incomplete, invalid, or inadequate evaluation can result in failure to identify reversible forms of dementia and in mistreatment and mismanagement. Of prime importance in the diagnosis of dementia in the elderly is to determine the cause, the course (whether the disease is fixed, likely to progress, or reversible), and the degree of disability as well as spared abilities. Until these determinations are made, treatment and management plans cannot be developed.

Of equal importance is that a diagnosis is too often made on the basis of a brief interview with the family members and a ten-minute mental status exam of the patient.

The purpose of this book is to help the diagnostician, clinicians, graduate students, health-care professionals, and family members understand causal factors, diagnostic procedures, and various treatment and management approaches.

The author has used the most current information available on the diagnosis, treatment, and management of Alzheimer's disease; however, medical sources and the advice of a physician are recommended regarding medical issues and diseases. Legal advice should be obtained from an attorney. The author does not claim to be a physician or attorney; and the advice given in this book is based on his training, education, and clinical experience as a licensed psychologist and doctor of psychology.

<hr>
<hr>

Prologue

Anna is a 67-year-old woman. Three years ago, her physician told her and her family that she was suffering from Alzheimer's disease. His diagnosis was based on a five-minute visit with the family and a ten minute examination of Anna. He observed that she was having problems with attention, concentration, and memory. He added that she also was "poorly oriented."

Following this visit to her physician, Anna's functional and cognitive abilities began to decline. A year later, she was placed in a nursing home. Her deterioration was so radical that the family requested public guardianship, stating that she often became nervous, had crying spells, and could not handle her affairs. It appears that her physician's diagnosis became a self-fulfilling prophecy.

About six months ago, a neurological assessment was requested. Following an extensive evaluation, it was determined that Anna was suffering from severe depression and generalized anxiety disorder. She was told that she did not have Alzheimer's disease. Another physician prescribed an antidepressant, and Anna began therapy. Today, Anna is living independently and is functional and relatively happy.

The misdiagnosis by her physician (based on lack of knowledge and use of inadequate assessment procedures) caused Anna and her family significant suffering and pain. It is the opinion of this author, based on many years of experience in the diagnosis of dementia and other psychopathologies in the elderly, that Anna's case is not unusual or uncommon.

This book is written with the hope that it will improve diagnostic methods and procedures as well as provide a basic understanding of Alzheimer's disease and other dementias in the elderly.

PART I

INTRODUCTION

CHAPTER 1

======

The Importance of a
Valid Diagnosis

Just a line to say I'm living,
  That I'm not among the dead;
Though I'm getting more forgetful,
  And more 'mixed up' in my head;
For, sometimes, I can't remember,
  Then I stand at foot of stair,
If I must go up for something,
  Or I've just come down from there,
And before the frig' so often,
  My poor mind is filled with doubt,
Have I just put food away, or
  Have I come to take some out,
And there's times when it is dark out,
  With my night cap on my head,
I don't know if I'm retiring,
  Or just getting out of bed,
So, if it's my turn to write you,
  There's no need in getting sore,
I may think I have written,
  And don't want to be a bore,
So, remember—I do love you,
  And wish that you were here;
But now it's nearly mail time,
  So I must say "Good-bye, dear",
There I stood beside the mailbox,
  With my face so very red,
Instead of mailing you my letter,
  I opened it instead.
                —Author unknown

Is this amusing poem an example of early stage Alzheimer's disease or symptomatic of age-associated memory impairment (AAMI)? As we age, we tend to have more problems with retrieval of information. AAMI differs from Alzheimer's in that retrieval or recall is improved when the individual is given time to, in effect, "search" the data bank. Cues also tend to improve memory in such situations. In the case of Alzheimer's, memory is not improved with cues or time.

Other symptoms and problems associated with Alzheimer's disease include aphasia (language disturbance); apraxia (inability to carry out motor tasks even though motor abilities are intact); agnosia (problems in recognizing or naming objects); and disturbances in such areas as abstraction, planning, and organizing. Sometimes there are also personality changes with irritability, anger, and aggressive acting out.

Yet many other disorders (physical and emotional) can present symptoms similar to Alzheimer's disease. Problems with concentration and attention as well as abstraction are common with mood disorders such as major depression. Individuals who have suffered from an ischemic or cardiovascular accident often have problems with reasoning and language. With Huntington's disease, there are commonly symptoms of attention disorder and behavioral problems. Medications can cause confusion, disorientation, and agitation.

The following case histories illustrate problems in proper diagnosis. All four of the individuals present symptoms of Alzheimer's; and in all four cases, the diagnosis was indeed Alzheimer's. Three of these diagnoses are inaccurate. In two of the cases, the disorders can be treated and the symptoms reversed. In a third illustration, dementia is present. However, the disorder is not progressive; and the management approach should be quite different than in the case of Alzheimer's disease.

CASE #1: MARIE

Marie is a 70-year-old white female who was admitted to a nursing home following surgery for a broken hip. Prior to admission to the facility, she had fallen on the ice. At the time of her evaluation, she had been a resident for about a week. Staff reported that she had adapted quite well to the home and had been friendly and cooperative. However, she spent most of her time in her room and did not interact with the other residents.

Medical problems, other than a broken hip, included hypertension and anemia. The individual had also been diagnosed as suffering from Alzheimer's disease. Family reported that the woman had become "forgetful and confused." At the time of the neuropsychological assessment, she was taking a major tranquilizer (neuroleptic) and an antianxiety drug.

During the evaluation, the subject was alert yet displayed a high level of anxiety and concern about her mental abilities. Mood was moderately depressed, with signs of disorientation and confusion. Visual and auditory abilities were adequate; and the subject was able to recall data regarding her family and her life situation, although retrieval was slow. Often she had to be cued to remember data and to express herself. On occasion, she had problems finding the correct word or words.

She knew the names of her four children and information regarding her recent accident. She also stated that her husband had died eight years ago from cancer and that she was "very sad." She said that problems in "finding the right words" resulted in embarrassment and that, for this reason, she did not want to interact with other residents.

During the testing, the individual displayed problems with orientation, registration, and expressive language. She also had problems with visual spatial motor tasks. She writes with a tremor and was unable to complete a sentence and copy geometric designs. This failure was due to motor deficit problems as well as visual spatial conceptual and perceptual problems. Judgment, reasoning, and reality testing were intact. She was able to learn new information as well as assimilate this information into a meaningful whole. She could read words and sentences but not numbers. Her responses to the self-report depression questionnaire indicate that she is moderately to severely depressed.

Prior to the neuropsychological assessment, the individual was diagnosed as suffering from "dementia." It is true that she presents many of the symptoms of Alzheimer's, including problems with expressive language (aphasia), problems with visual spatial motor tasks (apraxia), disorientation and confusion, and withdrawal. However, her problems are not progressive as in the case of Alzheimer's. She was able to learn new information, abstract, and reason. The proper diagnosis is vascular dementia and major depression, moderate to severe. The depression is related to unresolved grief about the death of her husband and concerns about her physical and mental health and about the future. There are specific focal impairments, however, and are very different from the impairments common among Alzheimer's patients. Unless there is another organic brain injury, it is probable that her abilities will improve. Alleviation of depression and anxiety tend to reduce problems with attention, concentration, and cognition. Functional abilities should also improve.

Recommendations given in this particular case included (1) discussion with the resident of her problems and concerns as well as unresolved losses and life situations. Assurance that she is not suffering from Alzheimer's is important. (2) Family involvement is primary to provide her with support and encouragement. (3) Speech and physical therapy, as well as social involvement, were suggested. (4) An antidepressant medication might be of benefit for a short time to lift her mood. Antianxiety medication is usually not prescribed in such cases in that it can be habit forming, can increase cognitive problems, and can cause paradoxical excitement.

This case is an example of an inaccurate diagnosis. The diagnosis Alzheimer's not only would rule out benefits from therapy to treat physical and emotional problems but also creates a sense of hopelessness and despair not only for the individual but also the family. With therapy and treatment of her medical condition and problems it is probable that she can return to live in a less structured and more autonomous and independent situation. (See the following chapters on types and levels of independent living options.)

CASE #2: MARY

Mary is a 78-year-old female who was living with her daughter prior to a fall about two years ago. At that time, she was admitted to a nursing home. Recently, she became very agitated, withdrawn, confused, and disoriented. She also had problems with memory and no longer participated in many of the activities which she had found enjoyable. Concern was expressed that she was suffering from Alzheimer's disease.

The individual was an attractive lady who was neatly and appropriately dressed. She was alert and oriented; however, there were signs of problems with concentration and some confusion regarding dates.

During the clinical interview, the woman expressed concern about her physical health. She stated that she had severe back pains. She continued that this pain decreased but that she was currently experiencing pain in her right arm. She added that she had recently decided "not to walk" and used a wheelchair. She said that this decision was not related to physical pain or fear of falling. When asked again why she did not walk, although physically able, she replied, "Well, I just decided not to walk."

The subject was also vague when asked about her withdrawal from activities. Until very recently, she enjoyed cards, bingo, and road trips. She was not suffering from auditory or visual problems. It appeared that her withdrawal was voluntary. She said that in the past she enjoyed playing the organ in the dining room but no longer had the ability. The subject stated that she had recently been "thinking" about the death of her husband almost a year before she entered the nursing home and about "how happy" she had been in the past.

The subject did very well on the tests and procedures of the neuropsychological assessment. (These tests and procedures, as well as the reason why a complete evaluation is necessary and of benefit, are discussed in detail in Chapter 14.) She was able to recall the date and provide information regarding the facility. There were no problems with attention, concentration, or recall. Remote, intermediate, and immediate memory were intact. There were no signs of psychosis or acute organicity. She did well on the tests that measure expressive and receptive language ability. She had some problems with tasks involving fine motor skills due to a tremor; however, visual spatial conceptual abilities were intact. Some anxiety was noted, with the probability that the anxiety did tend to impair task completion to some extent.

Initially, she denied that she was depressed; however, her score on the tests that measure mood disorders and her comments to this examiner, once rapport was established, resulted in the diagnosis major depression, severe. When talking about the death of her husband about three years earlier, she began to cry. She stated that she missed her home, her independence, her friends, and her role as a wife and community leader. She admitted that she was lonely and felt hopeless and helpless.

Major depression can cause symptoms such as withdrawal, lack of the ability to attend and concentrate, confusion, and anhedonia. In this case, it is probable that the woman focused on her physical problems initially as a new resident and that, at the time of testing, she was beginning to deal with her grief and depression as related to losses and her life-stage situation. Without an in-depth evaluation of cognitive, emotional, and functional abilities, her depression probably would not have been diagnosed or treated. The dementia-like symptoms would increase, and her functional and cognitive abilities would decrease. Fortunately, based on the assessment, she did receive treatment for her depression and is currently living a more satisfied and happy life.

It is significant that most elderly individuals are not adequately evaluated or treated for mental illness or problems until they are admitted to a nursing or medical facility. Unfortunately, mental illnesses are often ignored or denied. Family members tend to overlook the symptoms of mental illness, including the symptoms of Alzheimer's and other forms of dementia, until the individual suffering from the disorder becomes severely impaired and dysfunctional. Failure to diagnose and treat mental illness tends to increase pathology and suffering (see Soukup 1995).

CASE #3: SUE

The subject is an 86-year-old woman who was admitted to a nursing home about eighteen months prior to the assessment. On admission to the facility, she had reportedly been disoriented, confused, anxious, and agitated. Recently, behavioral problems had increased. Reportedly, she was more anxious and began wandering. Neuroleptic medication had been prescribed to alleviate anxiety and agitation; however, the improvement was minimal.

The subject was anxious and suspicious during the assessment. Rapport was not easily established. She had problems following simple directions and completing tasks that required more than one or two steps. She was able to answer some questions, though often confabulated. At times, she lost focus. Often directions, commands, and questions had to be repeated. Her medical record stated that there was no history of cardiovascular problems but that she suffered from hypertension. The second diagnosis was Alzheimer's disease.

During the clinical interview, the subject was unable to identify the date or provide significant life-situation data. She did not know how many children she had or where she had lived prior to admission to the home. She did know the day and month of her birth but was unable to recall the year or give an estimation of her age. She could not recall what she had for breakfast. When asked about her involvement in activities in the home she said, "I do whatever they do."

The individual had problems with orientation. She also displayed problems with attention and concentration. She was able to copy some of the geometric designs yet could not write her name or a sentence. She could read words and sentences but could not explain the meaning of the sentences or words.

The ability to plan, organize, and complete tasks was severely impaired, although some of the basic language skills had been spared. As is often the case in such situations, the individual appears more functional and able than in actuality. The ability to learn new information was severely impaired, which results in problems in adapting to new situations. Individuals with impaired memory and adaptive abilities often become confused and decompensate. Their confusion and frustration is a causal factor in their anxiety, agitation, and acting out.

The diagnosis in this case is dementia of the Alzheimer's type with behavioral disturbance and senile onset. At the time of the neuropsychological assessment, she was in middle- to late-stage Alzheimer's. (The progressive nature and various stages are discussed in Chapters 2 and 17). Recommendations for management included providing stability and consistency in the environment; limiting stimulation; limiting decisions and choices required; continued family involvement with family possibly benefiting from an Alzheimer's support group; and use of cuing, repetition, and demonstration in communicating with the individual. More is presented on management and communication techniques in dealing with individuals suffering from Alzheimer's in Chapters 19 and 21.

CASE #4: DOROTHY

The subject in this assessment is a 74-year-old female who had been diagnosed as suffering from hypertension, arterial sclerotic heart disease, arthritis, and Alzheimer's disease. She, too, was in a nursing home. The diagnoses were made by her physician. Staff at the nursing home reported a number of odd and bizarre behaviors. Allegedly, the woman continually washes and rewashes her clothes. Following meals, she strips to her undergarments and scrubs herself with alcohol or soap, or at least attempts to do this. Usually staff stops her. Also, the individual continually cleans her room. According to staff, her compulsions interfere with her functional ability. She refuses to enter into social activities or participate in physical therapy because, in the words of staff, "she is too busy cleaning things." When tested, the individual was sitting in a reclining chair in her room. She was barefoot. Grooming and hygiene were marginal. She was alert, cooperative, and very verbal. She enjoyed talking about herself and her life.

There were some signs of cognitive problems. She lacked focus and often became tangential and circumstantial. However, there were no signs of hallucinations. Hearing was moderately impaired. (Speech, hearing, and vision problems in the elderly tend to result in problems with comprehending the environment. Often, individuals with these disabilities become withdrawn. Communication and comprehension problems often lead to confusion, frustration, and irritability. It is not uncommon for individuals with these disabilities to be diagnosed as demented.) This particular individual admitted to hearing problems. She said that she had hearing aids yet refused to wear them.

Mental abilities appeared to be in the average range. There were some signs of problems with attention and concentration; however, testing indicated that this probably was due to lack of interest and motivation, the fact that she was in her own obsessive–compulsive world, and her emotional state. Referral to her social history provided information that she has abused alcohol for years. As is discussed in Chapter 3, alcohol abuse can result in a number of cognitive problems, including problems with memory, expressive language, and abstract reasoning.

This case presented the examiner with a diagnostic problem. There were symptoms of memory and orientation problems, confusion, and odd and bizarre thought process. However, was the individual suffering from Alzheimer's; the residual effects of alcohol abuse; psychosis; or some other form of psychopathology, vascular dementia, toxicity due to medication, or a characterological disorder?

Extensive testing using both neuropsychological and psychological techniques and instruments resulted in the diagnosis of major depres-

sion, severe recurrent and obsessive–compulsive disorder. It was determined that she acted in strange and unusual ways but was not psychotic. Her problems with task completion, especially tasks involving
visual motor skills, were related to chronic and static organicity as
well as lack of interest and attention. Expressive language ability was
intact, which helps rule out organicity due to alcohol abuse. However,
reasoning was very concrete. This suggests lack of natural endowment,
enrichment, or education.

The responses to the self-report depression rating inventory and
scale, as well as comments made during the clinical interview, reflect
severe depression. The individual internalizes a great deal of shame,
guilt, and self-hatred. She stated that she had suicidal ideations in the
past and had been under care for depression. Her depression was related to having a child out of wedlock, the death of another child in a
fire, alcoholism, extramarital affairs, and legal problems. She stated
that during her early and middle adult years, she cleaned houses for a
living. From a psychodynamic standpoint, her compulsion to clean is
an attempt to "clean herself" and eliminate the feelings of guilt and
self-hatred.

Recommendations made in this case included the following:

1. Consideration of psychotropic medication to alleviate depression and control obsessive–compulsive behavior
2. Psychotherapy to explore feelings of guilt, self-hatred, and failure
3. A hearing evaluation
4. Encouraging the individual to become more actively involved socially and
   to develop interests other than cleaning
5. Involvement of family to explore the past; improve communication; build
   acceptance and hope for forgiveness; and resolve some of the issues that
   have caused this woman feelings of guilt, depression, and anxiety

These cases illustrate the need for an accurate and complete diagnosis. All four of the individuals had been diagnosed as suffering from
Alzheimer's. The standard treatment in Alzheimer's is to calm the
patient and provide for the individual's physical and hygienic needs.
In three of the four cases presented, the individuals were not suffering
from Alzheimer's and needed much more than merely caring for their
health and physical needs.

The following chapters discuss Alzheimer's disease, additional psychological and physical disorders which present as Alzheimer's, and
other forms of dementia. Some of these dementias are reversible and
treatable. This is also discussed.

CHAPTER 2

Dementia of the Alzheimer's Type:
Prevalence, Symptoms,
Course, and Case Studies

I used to play bridge and write poetry.
Now I don't even know my grandchildren's names.
—Comment during clinical interview with
middle-stage Alzheimer's patient

The Diagnostic and Statistical Manual of Mental Disorders, Fourth Edition *(DSM-IV)* defines dementia as a disorder resulting in cognitive impairments and due to physiological conditions. Symptoms are sufficiently severe to significantly impair social and functional abilities. The disturbances are emotional, cognitive, and behavioral. Specific cognitive impairments can include memory problems; aphasia; apraxia; agnosia; and problems with planning, organizing, and abstract reasoning.

Problems with memory are debilitating because inability to encode, store, and retrieve new information limits adaptive skills as well as task completion. Individuals commonly have trouble completing projects or simple functions which require more than one step. Making coffee in the morning becomes a difficult task because the person suffering from dementia has lost the ability to sequence and move from one step to another. Memory problems also frequently result in interpersonal problems. The victim of Alzheimer's disease tends to ask the same question repeatedly. This is because they are unable to remember that they asked the question. Alzheimer's sufferers also tend to become angry and irritable when they misplace items of significance. Paranoia and suspiciousness are common.

Language disturbance makes expression of wishes and needs difficult and can lead to frustration and misunderstanding. Receptive language defects with inability to understand spoken or written
statements and commands further impair functional ability. Apraxia
can result in impaired ability to carry out simple self-care tasks such
as combing one's hair or getting dressed. Individuals suffering from
dementia often have problems recognizing family members or even
their own reflection in the mirror. Tactile senses may also be impaired
where the patient cannot recognize such items as keys or coins by touch.
As the dementia progresses or in cases such as vascular dementia
affecting the frontal lobe, disturbances in executive functioning tend
to take place. Impaired abstract reasoning results in an inability to
make logical decisions and judgments and to problem solve. Reality
testing becomes impaired. Often, there are personality changes with
the risk of aggressive or assaultive behaviors. These responses are related to a lack of impulse control, as well as frustration and confusion,
due to lack of comprehension of one's environment and situational
factors. Individuals suffering from dementia are frequently disoriented
as to place, time, and person. Disturbance of gait is an associated feature of dementia, which carries with it the risk of falling. Inappropriate social and sexual behavior and anxiety are additional associated
features, as are sleep, appetite, and mood disturbances. Because individuals with dementia are more likely to be impacted by change, physical stressors (such as illness or surgery) and psychological stress can
create radical mood disturbances. Delusions, hallucinations, and delirium are also associated features of dementia.

PREVALENCE AND COURSE

According to *DSM-IV*, the age of onset of dementia depends on the
type. However, dementia commonly takes place late in life. It is estimated that from 2 to 4 percent of the population over age 65 have
dementia of the Alzheimer's type. The prevalence of Alzheimer's in
individuals over age 85 runs from 20 to 25 percent. It is estimated that
50 percent of individuals in nursing homes suffer from dementia.
However, as is discussed later, this may be an exaggeration because of
inaccurate and inadequate testing and assessment procedures and
practices. *DSM-IV* states that an assessment should include not only a
mental status examination but also a neuropsychological assessment.

Originally, dementia was imaged as a progressive process with continual deterioration in functional and cognitive ability. While
Alzheimer's disease is progressive, other forms are not necessarily
progressive. Dementia can be progressive, static, or remitting. About

50 percent of the dementias are considered treatable or reversible. This is why an accurate diagnosis and treatment plan is essential. In Chapter 1, the dementia illustrated in Case #1 is related to a cardiovascular accident. Unless there are additional injuries or insults, the disabilities and impairments should remain at the current level or remit. Marie can be taught new skills; and, with help, her confusion and problems with memory should improve. In Case #2, Mary suffers from depression, which can be treated by pharmacological and psychotherapeutic means. Sue (Case #3) suffers from Alzheimer's. This is not reversible; however, her agitation, anxiety, and behavior can be managed and her quality of life maintained to some degree. Focus on health and hygiene needs will be of primary importance. The prognosis is for a continued deterioration with a vegetative state likely unless death occurs first. (It is estimated that the average life of an individual with Alzheimer's is eight to ten years from onset. Physical deterioration tends to lag cognitive and functional deterioration.) Dorothy (Case #4) is suffering from depression and obsessive–compulsive disorder. Again, once identified, this disorder can be treated.

Alzheimer's disease is the most common of the dementias. The course of the disease is progressive, with the onset insidious. Early deficits include recent memory, followed by problems in orientation, language, and abstract thinking. During the early stages, there is usually a recognition of lost capacities and abilities with expressed concern and anxiety. However, individuals commonly attempt to "cover up" their disabilities and problems. They tend to confabulate and deny their problems to others. Family members are usually in denial, looking for and hoping for an improvement in ability and cognition. Unfortunately, family denial only postpones adequate assessment and professional help.

As the disorder progresses, problems develop in social and occupational areas. If the individual is still working, co-workers may be aware of the individual's poor performance. The sufferer may have problems in remembering names and may become confused or lost. Anxiety is common during this stage.

With time, individuals with Alzheimer's disease fail to recognize familiar faces; develop problems with attention, concentration, and simple task completion; have difficulty traveling alone to familiar places; and tend to withdraw. During late-stage Alzheimer's, incontinence is common, with severe disorientation. Often the individual becomes mute and bedridden, unable to perform basic self-care tasks.

Emotional responses during the cycle commonly include confusion, anxiety, and depression during the early stage; irritability, anger, and inappropriate acting out during the middle stage; and withdrawal and vegetation in late-stage dementia. The level of agitation and acting out tends to be related to premorbid personality traits, although this is not always true.

Alzheimer's disease can be early onset (65 years of age or younger) or late onset (over age 65). Late onset is more common. Early onset used to be referred to as presenile dementia, with late onset identified as senile dementia. Subtypes of Alzheimer's include dementia of the Alzheimer's type with delirium, with delusions, with depressed mood, uncomplicated, and with behavioral disturbances. Behavioral disturbances are most common in middle-stage Alzheimer's as the patient becomes more confused, disoriented, and dysfunctional. It is interesting that depression is most common in early-stage Alzheimer's. As the disorder progresses, the patient tends to become less aware of the specific nature of the losses and more irritable, oppositional, and dysphoric.

CASE #5: CAROL

Middle-Stage Dementia of the Alzheimer's Type

The subject is a 94-year-old woman who was tested in an intensive care facility, where she had lived for about four years. Prior to that time, she had resided in a congregate care setting. Transfer to the nursing home was related to a deterioration in ability to care for herself. A neuropsychological assessment was ordered to determine the level of disability and make management and care recommendations. The individual had been diagnosed as suffering from arthritis and hypertension. Caretakers stated that she displayed radical mood swings and often becomes angry and agitated. She no longer appeared to be aware of cognitive problems or depressed by losses in memory and functional ability. Staff reported that the subject still recognizes family members and is pleased by their visits. However, she usually does not interact with them.

During the testing, it was determined that she has severe expressive and receptive language deficits. Attention and concentration were limited. She had problems understanding directions and following simple instructions and commands. At times, she became incoherent and agitated; however, she appeared to enjoy the attention provided her. Immediate, short-term, and remote memory were impaired. She answered many questions with the responses "Yes" or "I don't know." She was unable to recall what she had for breakfast or information about the facility. She did not know the day of the year, month, or season. (This is common with elderly patients in an intensive care facility. Temporal data are not of great interest or significance.) She did not know the names of her adult children or her deceased husband.

The subject did poorly on the mental status exam. She was unable to repeat words and simple phrases. She was also unable to complete a three-stage task, although she did close her eyes on command. Cuing, repetition, and demonstration did improve performance to some extent; however, she was unable to assimilate new information and knowledge. She was able to read some words and sentences but did poorly on the abstract thinking and complex ideation tests. (These tests and tasks are discussed in Chapter 14.) The subject also did poorly on the Boston Aphasia Test and the Boston Naming Test, indicating that she suffers from agnosia and aphasia. These are symptoms of middle-stage dementia of the Alzheimer's type, which is the correct diagnosis in this case.

It is significant that the individual was able to answer some questions and perform some tasks such as reading words and sentences. Without a complete assessment, one would tend to overestimate the individual's abilities and functional skills. This evaluation was important in that a more accurate determination of spared skills and abilities as well as impairments was provided. The individual cannot learn new information and thus has problems in adapting to new and changing conditions. Thus, a recommendation was made to provide stability and consistency. The individual tended to become confused and overstimulated; thus, stimulation should be limited. Family members were advised to keep visits short, with a minimal number of visitors at one time. The subject had problems understanding conversations and commands; so caretakers must be specific, direct, and concrete in interactions. Cuing demonstration and repetition were recommended. Expressive language skills are poor, so family and staff must attempt to anticipate the patient's needs. Active listening is necessary.

The individual is still fairly physically able and needs some form of physical activity, even though her actions are no longer goal directed. The patient also responds to attention and needs touching and love. It was suggested that family members might just be with the resident, hold her hand, and listen to music. Making demands on an individual who is in middle-stage Alzheimer's or expecting them to carry on a conversation often results in agitation, anxiety, and dysphoria.

CASE #6: HELEN

Late-Stage Dementia of the Alzheimer's Type

Helen is 89 years old. She had been in a nursing home for seven years when tested. Her medical history indicated that she suffers from dehydration, diabetes, congestive heart failure, and coronary artery disease. She also had been diagnosed as suffering from "organic brain syndrome," which is nonspecific and gives little indication as to the nature of her dementia and level of competency and functional ability.

At the time of testing, the individual was in a stupor; however, when observed later in the day, she became restless and agitated. Staff reported that she tends to be very disoriented and, on occasion, combative. Expressive language abilities were very limited, as was the ability to carry out tasks and respond to commands. She did respond to auditory and tactile stimulation and was able to track visually. The diagnosis of late-stage dementia of the Alzheimer's type was provisional because many of the assessment procedures and tasks could not be administered or completed by the subject. In this case, it appears that cognitive and functional abilities will not improve and that the focus of treatment should be on medical problems and in making the patient as comfortable as possible. In similar cases of agitation, anxiety, and combativeness, a low dosage of a high-potency neuroleptic on an as-needed (prn) basis has been used successfully.

Cases #5 and #6 have been included to illustrate the progressive and nonreversible nature of Alzheimer's. Because the disease is so debilitating and dehumanizing and because of the impact on family members, the disorder is greatly feared. Research indicates that the prevalence of Alzheimer's is increased in individuals with Down's syndrome and in individuals with a history of head injuries. The disorder is more common among females than males. This might be related to the fact that females tend to live longer than males and that late-onset Alzheimer's is more common than early-onset Alzheimer's.

Laboratory findings show that specific brain atrophy is present in Alzheimer's with wider cortical sulci and cerebral ventricles than in normal same-age individuals. Neuroimaging may aid in a differential diagnosis of the various dementias. However, behavioral observations are more specific as far as deficits and impairments are concerned and offer more information as to the cause, the course, and treatment and management techniques and possibilities.

CHAPTER 3

Other Forms of Dementia
Affecting the Elderly

Age is a state of mind.
Do not regret growing old.
It is a privilege denied many.
———Author unknown

Of course the "privilege" is not as great or enjoyable when one is physically or mentally impaired or disabled.

The second most common form of dementia affecting the elderly is vascular dementia (see Case #1 [Chapter 1]). This used to be called multi-infarct dementia. The cognitive impairments present are similar to those associated with Alzheimer's disease. These include memory impairment as well as one or more of the following: aphasia, apraxia, agnosia, or disturbance of executive functions. There must be a significant impairment in social or occupational functioning and a significant decline in abilities from a previous level, as well as evidence of cerebrovascular disease either from laboratory evidence or based on neurological symptoms. Subtypes include the following: with delirium, with delusions, with depressed mood, uncomplicated, and with behavioral disturbance. Thus, the symptoms and subtypes of Alzheimer's-type dementia are alike; however, the difference is that in vascular dementia, there is evidence of a cardiovascular accident (CVA) or transient ischemic attack (TIA). The course and treatment of the two forms of dementia also vary radically. The prognosis for Alzheimer's patients is poor, with continued deterioration of abilities. Patients who are suffering from vascular dementia do not face a deterioration of ability unless there is additional injury or insult. In some cases, impairments and disabilities will actually become less severe, especially with medical treatment. Another difference is that with vascular dementia the onset is typically abrupt, followed by a fluctuating course. Also, the impairment is usually specific and corresponds with the part of the brain that has been damaged. Paralysis, motor function deficits, and expressive language deficits are common. In vascular dementia, there is also an element of prevention which is not possible with Alzheimer's. Treatment of hypertension and vascular disease can reduce risk of a CVA with the related damage to the brain.

The onset of vascular dementia tends to be earlier than that of Alzheimer's. Vascular dementia is more common among males than females. Use of computerized tomography (CT) and magnetic resonance imaging (MRI) tends to lead to detection of vascular dementia based on an abnormal amount or extent of central nervous system lesions. While there is evidence of senile plaques, neurofibrillary tangles, neuronal loss, and granulovascular degeneration with Alzheimer's disease, the difference between the normal aging brain and the Alzheimer's patient is not significant.

DSM-IV also identifies dementias related to general medical conditions, substance-induced persisting dementias, dementias due to multiple etiologies, and dementias not otherwise specified. These dementias present symptoms similar to Alzheimer's; however, the course of the dementia and treatment is quite different. Again, this emphasizes the importance of a complete evaluation of the individual. A history, physical examination, or laboratory finding is required to classify a dementia as related to a general condition.

It is important to distinguish between reversible dementia and those which are not. Symptoms of major depression often include problems with concentration, attention, and memory; disturbance of executive functions and impaired reasoning, judgment, and reality testing. Major depression is treatable (see Case #2); and, like the following disorders and diseases, the related dementia symptoms are partially or fully reversible. In some of the disorders, brain damage cannot be reversed; however, impairments can be remediated to some extent. Individuals who suffer from schizophrenia also have problems with concentration, organization of thoughts, reality testing, expressive language, and communication. In some forms of schizophrenia (catatonic and disorganized), there may be mutism and a near-vegetative state similar to late-stage Alzheimer's.

CASE #7: CLARA

This individual has a history of psychiatric hospitalizations. When tested, she was 83 years old. It was reported that she was displaying radical mood swings and was paranoid. Auditory hallucinations and asocial personality traits were also reported. On occasion, the individual allegedly became verbally abusive to family and friends.

At the time of testing, she was appropriately dressed and alert. She was cooperative and friendly, except for one occasion, when she became very angry and agitated without known cause. She was obviously responding to internal stimuli. Her mood was moderately elevated with symptoms of hypomania. She was not actively psychotic but did admit to hallucinations in the past. Thought processes were poorly focused, with a tendency to become circumstantial. Memory and orientation were moderately impaired. These symptoms of memory impairment, problems with attention and concentration, and mood lability are similar to those associated with Alzheimer's. However, there were significant differences in ability in this case as compared to the impairments common to Alzheimer's patients. This individual scored in the normal range on the mental status exam. She was able to complete complicated tasks and follow directions accurately. She also was not suffering from aphasia or agnosia. Most significant, she was able to comprehend and assimilate new information. There were signs of paranoia; however, these appear to be chronic and characterological rather than related to organic causes. She also showed signs of depression. Individuals with Alzheimer's are often sad and anxious rather than depressed. Based on past history, her medical records, interviews with family, and the neuropsychological assessment, she was diagnosed as suffering from schizoaffective disorder. Recommendations include consideration of antidepressant and neuroleptic medication; elimination of anxiety-producing situations, with caretakers being nonconfrontive whenever possible; stability and structure in her environment and life; and psychological and psychiatric treatment as required based on monitoring her mood and behavior. There existed the possibility for another psychotic episode.

A number of drugs, both prescription and nonprescription, have cognitive impairing side effects. Often, they have a synergetic impact. This is why it is important to monitor the drugs used by elderly patients. Dementia syndromes can develop from the use of benzodiazepines, barbiturates, stimulants, and some neuroleptic medications. This is discussed more fully in Chapters 3 and 17.

Alcohol, inhalants, hypnotics, and anxiolytics can also cause cognitive impairment. However, in these cases, the dementia is usually acute with remission over a period of time following abstinence. Response to some of these drugs is usually delirium or acute psychosis, in the case of hallucinogens, rather than dementia-like symptoms. However, drug toxicity possibilities must be ruled out when diagnosing Alzheimer's.

Metabolic disorders can also cause dementia-like symptoms. Azotemia usually produces impaired concentration, low energy, and irritability. Hypoglycemia tends to present as delirium in severe cases. Liver failure can result in clouded sensorium and mental dullness. Thyroid disease is associated with problems in thinking, lethargy, slowed speech, and impaired memory. Hypercalcemia often has similar side effects. Cushing's syndrome can cause depression and delirium. Infection and fever in the elderly may be causal factors in cognitive impairment. Pneumonia, urinary tract infections and generalized sepsis are the most common infections in the elderly population. Vitamin deficiencies and poor diet can result in sensorial impairment and problems with attention, concentration, and reasoning.

Other dementias listed in *DSM-IV* include dementia due to human immunodeficiency virus (HIV); head trauma; and Parkinson's, Huntington's, Pick's, and Creutzfeldt–Jakob diseases.

While this is just a partial list of the reversible dementias, it illustrates the need to be aware of possible medical causes of dementia. A physical exam, medical history, neurological exam, and blood and urine tests are often appropriate to rule out dementias due to other general medical conditions. A history of drug use and inventory might also be of value in the case of suspected organicity due to substance abuse or dependency.

CHAPTER 4

The Aging Process:
Normal and Successful Aging

CASE #8: DAN

Dan is 79 years old. He retired at age 58 from his career as an airline pilot. Since that time, he has continued an active and satisfying life. He walks with a quick gait and climbs on his roof to clean out the gutters. He is mentally alert and displays a sense of humor and a curiosity about life. He enjoys the outdoors and his male friends with whom he fishes and hunts. He owns his home as well as a vacation home in the north woods.

His time is spent repairing his home, fixing his car, and taking care of his wife. He is sociable and flirts with women of all ages, although his fidelity to his wife of fifty-five years is evident. He does not smoke. He drinks a glass or two of wine on occasion. Recently, he purchased a new car and attempted to have the warranty extended to ten years and 100,000 miles. He anticipates that he will outlast the car but still wants protection.

Dan has a positive outlook on life and the future. He has daily tasks and goals. He has no major physical problems and is fortunate in that he is financially secure. He has had tragedy in his life. A daughter died when she was 30 years old and left three small children. Also, his wife is recovering from a rather severe stroke. However, Dan has dealt with the hardships of life in an appropriate and adaptive way. He has resolved past losses and grief and looks at the future in a realistic and pragmatic way. He sees life with a certain detachment. Death is seen as inevitable but not feared.

Dan has been fortunate; he has not suffered from financial, emotional, or physical disabilities. His wife, on the other hand, is severely disabled because of a cardiovascular accident. Following the CVA, she could not speak or walk. With therapy, she has recovered her speech and can walk slowly but has weakness of the left side. She also has some memory problems. Thought processes are slow. She needs extra time to perform tasks that were relatively simple for her prior to the heart attack. She relies on her husband more and more, yet both resist placing her in a nursing facility. In the early years of their life and marriage, Dan's wife cared for the house and the family. Now the roles have reversed. Dan takes most of the responsibility, and his wife has become very dependent. However, it can be considered that Dan and his wife have aged successfully.

Successful aging tends to be correlated with physical and mental health, especially the continuation of cognitive ability and flexibility. The continued pursuit of interests and activities appears to be important in successful aging. Studies have also suggested that having a marital partner improves the level of happiness and satisfaction in late-stage life. Financial security tends to enhance adjustment in the aging process. Other factors include maintaining physical fitness and continuing to learn and stay involved socially.

The way that individuals interpret their lives and situation also appears to be important in successful aging as well as how they judge the future and their concept regarding death and dying. Elderly individuals tend to reminisce. A life review is often suggested as a way of resolving old issues and preserving a sense of identity and self-esteem. This process is discussed in Chapter 21.

Psychological aging and biological aging are quite different. Both are significant in the consideration of aging. Various forms of psychopathology are discussed in that they often present symptoms of dementia. Physical and medical problems are also discussed. Briefly, we review psychological development and the aging process with a focus on successful aging and then discuss the normal aging process from a physiological basis.

Erik Erikson (1980) is best known for his works related to successful psychosocial development during the life stage. He relates successful aging to the accomplishment of various tasks. Emotional problems develop, according to his paradigm, when these tasks are not completed. The last two stages of development are generativity versus stagnation and ego integrity versus despair. Generativity is the ability to show concern about the next generation and the future of society. Erikson would suggest that continued involvement with family and community adds to late-life enjoyment and satisfaction. Caring for grandchildren, teaching, and being involved in worthwhile community projects are a few ways of fulfilling one's obligation and staying invested. Stagnation is, on the other hand, a tendency to be egocentric, self-involved, and self-indulgent.

Ego integrity suggests a satisfaction with one's life and coming to a sense of acceptance. It implies forgiveness and resolution of negative issues with feelings of self-worth, accomplishment, and well-being. Despair is often signaled by fear of death and feelings of anger, dissatisfaction, and isolation. Dan and his wife appear to have accomplished their goals and live a life of relative satisfaction and happiness.

CASE #9: ROSE

Rose lives in a nursing home. She is 78 years old. Until about three years ago, she lived independently in a retirement facility. Most of her life, she has been isolated, suspicious, and angry. She has few friends and is withdrawn and distrustful. Since age 45, she has been unemployed. Problems with fellow employees led to termination. When assessed, she was in a wheelchair because of osteoarthritis. Vision is impaired; however, she refuses to be evaluated for corrective glasses. As she states, "What's the use? It won't help." Hearing is intact. Her husband died about ten years ago. She described her marriage as "bad." She continued, "But we stayed together because it was the thing to do."

The woman's daughter described her as "mean spirited," adding that she has "always been verbally abusive to everyone in the family." Rose complained that none of her two adult children or grandchildren visit her. She said, "My son comes once a week to bring me my laundry and stays for twenty minutes." Rose has few contacts with the other residents at the nursing home. She explained, "They are all too nosy. I'd rather just stay in my room." Rose has not aged successfully.

Robert Peck (1968) suggests that there are three psychological adjustments in later life which are important to successful aging. The first is ego differentiation versus work role preoccupation. Many individuals identify so strongly with their work that as retirement draws near or in cases of job loss or role changes, they become depressed and lose a sense of self. Peck suggests that there are ways to remain involved and stay active and alert. Many individuals presenting with dementia in late adulthood are actually depressed. They have not adequately made the transition from a work-related identity to that of an individual who is valuable and valued because of other abilities and traits.

A second adjustment has to do with overcoming a preoccupation with the body and one's physical situation or condition. As is discussed in more depth later, aging results in such changes as loss of physical strength, muscle tone, and bone density. Pain is not uncommon due to arthritic conditions. However, individuals who have aged successfully tend to focus on the possibility of enjoying life with a sense transcendence. Rose focused on her physical problems and symptoms all her life with unfortunate results.

CASE #10: ANN

Ann is 88 years old. She is fragile and suffers from arthritis, congestive heart failure, and problems with hearing. She lives independently.
Her adult son and wife live a few blocks away from her. They call her
or stop in to see her two or three times a day. Ann drives her own car,
plays bridge with her bridge group, and bakes wonderful homemade
pies and biscuits which make her a valued guest at social gatherings
throughout the county. Although her pain is severe, she rarely talks
about it. About six months ago, she fell down on her front steps and
was unable to get up. She knew that her son would not be coming to
check on her for three or four more hours, and she did not carry an
emergency beeper as had been suggested. It was a crisp fall morning,
and it began to rain. After shouting for ten minutes, Ann said to herself, "Get up you old fool. You aren't hurt." With this, she dragged
herself up the steps and crawled into bed. Her son finally came to
check on her. Ann is now up and about, although she has to use a
walker. She still bakes the best biscuits in the county.

Peck concludes that the third primary psychological task is ego transcendence versus ego preoccupation. This is similar to Erikson's ego
integrity versus despair. Peck writes that this is coming to the realization that one will die. This stage or state is not a passive acceptance of
death but an adaptation requiring unselfish and generous living based
on the belief that one has lived successfully and will continue to share
in one's later years. Caring for another often helps. Spouses of
Alzheimer's patients often show a love and unselfishness which is
difficult for others to imagine or duplicate. It is not uncommon for the
caretaking spouse to live until the Alzheimer's patient dies and then
make his or her own transition.

Daniel Levinson (1978) refers to transition periods in life. He describes
four eras: (1) childhood adolescence, (2) early adulthood, (3) middle
adulthood, and (4) late adulthood. During late adulthood, Levinson
claims, there is often a fear of loss of physical potency and grieving
about lost abilities and capacities. This often results in the severe depression which is found among the elderly. On the other hand, others
see late adulthood as a time of fewer responsibilities and a time for leisure and pleasure. Ann and Dan have been successful because they
have focused on the joy of living rather than the fear of aging and death.

The preceding information has been related to psychological aging
with an emphasis on successful aging and how attitude and outlook
on life can influence happiness and satisfaction. This section focuses
on the physiological biological aging process.

Aging is a process from conception to death. Among humans, there
is a vast difference in the rate of aging and the type and degree of
disability during the deterioration process. After age 50 or 55, there is

commonly a decline in physical vigor and health; however, some individuals have little decline until the 70s. Organs also age at different rates. Teeth and eyes tend to show signs of deterioration sooner than other parts of the body.

Scientists have suggested that collagen, the material that supports the cells of the body, often becomes hard and brittle during the aging process and that this is significant in disease with a decreasing ability to ward off insults to the body. Studies suggest that after about age 30, collagen begins to become more brittle.

Muscular changes in the body are also related to health. The body consists of striped or voluntary muscles that control motor movement and involuntary or smooth muscles that are found in the intestines, stomach wall, blood vessels, and most of the internal organs. Muscle strength tends to decline after age 25 to 30. There is also a loss of elasticity, although exercise can delay these losses and decline.

Bone loss of size and strength takes place in both sexes but at a faster rate among females. Arthritis tends to begin after age 40. Research suggests that emotional factors can be a contributing factor. Rose (Case #9), who suffers from severe arthritis, has been an angry, negative, vindictive person all her life.

More than two-thirds of the individuals over age 75 have dentures. This rate appears to be decreasing with better hygiene and more emphasis on care. Loss of teeth can be a real problem in the elderly. Adequate nutrition is dependent on the ability to eat a variety of foods. It is not uncommon to find malnutrition and disease related to poor diet in the elderly, especially those living alone who are suffering from some form of dementia or functional disability.

Problems with mobility are common as one ages due to loss of bone content as well as muscle atrophy. Paralysis due to a CVA or TIA is more likely as one advances in age. Parkinson's disease causes problems with gait, equilibrium, and balance. Cramps and stiffness can increase with age.

The cardiovascular system changes with age. While the heart tends to maintain its size, tissue atrophy takes place and arteries lose elasticity. Hardening and shrinkage of the arteries decrease blood flow. The heart works harder as a result of hardening and shrinkage of the arteries, increasing the possibility of CVA. Disease of the heart is the number-one cause of death in individuals over age 65, followed by malignant neoplasms, cardiovascular disease, pneumonia, and arteriosclerosis.

Respiratory problems cause a decrease in the oxygen the blood receives and that is available for dispersement to the body tissues and organs. After age 40, the basal metabolic rate declines gradually. After age 80, the decline is rapid. Speaking problems are common in the elderly, related not only to stroke but also to other factors. Voice timbre and quality change. Problems with expressive language can present as dementia. Hearing loss and deficits also increase problems in functioning, comprehension, and relating to others.

CASE #11: HENRY

Henry was 83 years old when tested for cognitive and functional problems. His medical records indicated that he suffered from a CVA and a number of TIAs. He was confined to a wheelchair. His family reported that he had problems with swallowing and often refused to eat. Recently, he had become more and more withdrawn. About four years prior to the time of the neuropsychological assessment, he had been tested for hearing loss and been provided with hearing aids for both ears. However, the family had not emphasized the importance of using them for a number of years. Not surprising, Henry was becoming less communicative and involved. A test of auditory ability determined that his hearing loss had gone from moderate to severe. With new hearing aids, he became much more involved and interested in the world around him. Memory, concentration, and attention improved. His depression also lifted.

Research indicates that changes take place in the central nervous system during aging with a reduction of blood (and thus oxygen) to the brain and cerebral atrophy. Causal factors in Alzheimer's and other forms of dementia are discussed in Chapters 6 and 16. One of the theories is that neuritic plaques and neurofibrillary tangles form with granulovascular degeneration.

The efficiency of the urinary system decreases with age, with incontinence becoming more common. Incontinence tends to have related emotional and psychological impact, with many of the elderly experiencing severe feelings of shame and inadequacy. Anger is also a common emotion. During aging, the kidney becomes less effective in removing toxins. This is one reason that medications should be closely monitored in the elderly.

The immune system tends to become less responsive and efficient with age. As an example of this, the mortality rate from pneumonia is six to seven times greater among the elderly than for young adults.

The preceding section on biological aging might be seen as bleak with the view that old age is a progressively degenerative process leading to pain, dysfunction, and disability. This is not so. Only 5 percent of the elderly population require intensive care prior to death. Many people live happy, successful, rich lives—like Dan and Ann. The elderly are not, as often portrayed, necessarily infirmed, dependent, and demented. Living life fully and developing a healthy attitude toward dying appear to present some benefits. Ethel Waters once said, "I'm not afraid to die. I kinda look forward to it. I know the Lord has His arms wrapped around this big fat sparrow."

CHAPTER 5

The Reversible Dementias versus the Irreversible Dementias

In the Prologue and Chapter 1, cases of misdiagnosed Alzheimer's disease were presented. Chapters 2 and 3 discussed *DSM-IV* criteria for Alzheimer's and other dementias. The importance of an adequate and accurate assessment, as well as the need to identify impaired and spared abilities and skills, was also discussed. This chapter focuses on the dementias that are reversible as opposed to the irreversible dementias.

Reversible dementias can be treated. Failure to diagnose reversible dementias results in failure to treat the disorder. Failure to treat, of course, results in failure to remediate the impairments and disabilities. The following cases are illustrations of a failure to recognize and treat the causes of disorders that result in cognitive and functional problems. Case #12 is one in which an individual was suffering from delusional (paranoid) disorder as well as depression. In Case #13, the individual is schizophrenic.

CASE #12: JOHN

John was 77 years old when he moved to a nursing home following a stroke. Before that time, he had lived with his wife. The stroke had left him partially paralyzed. He was unable to use his left hand or walk without assistance. In the past, prior to retirement, he had been a carpenter. He expressed a great deal of pride in his work and lamented the fact that he could no longer use his hands for woodworking.

His marriage of twenty-seven years was described as "good." However, later in the clinical interview, he stated that it was his belief that his wife was having an affair. She is 76 years old and his second wife. He also accused her of trying to steal his money. His distrust and suspiciousness appeared to be global with reports that his roommate had a gun and wanted to kill him. He added that the staff had "demons" on them and that someone had tied a bomb to his wheelchair.

This individual had not been properly diagnosed. The diagnostician had not taken a social history or adequately assessed the extent of the delusions and the cause. It was determined that the delusions were not related to dementia as diagnosed originally but were a form of regression and decompensation. The individual had maintained his cognitive abilities, with memory, language skills, attention, and abstract reasoning intact. His delusions were very specific and an indication of his feelings of powerlessness and helplessness. Neuroleptic medication was not the answer. He did respond to psychotherapy directed at alleviating his depression and improving his adaptation to the facility and an acceptance of his condition and situation. Prior to the assessment, his condition was considered to be untreatable and irreversible. Staff considered him just another angry, strange old man.

CASE #13: DON

Don has a history of schizophrenia. However, on admission to a nursing home, he was diagnosed as suffering from Alzheimer's disease. Staff said that he was disoriented and confused. His thought-processing problems were considered a form of dementia. However, they were very different from the symptoms of dementia. There were no signs of aphasia, apraxia, or agnosia. Memory was intact. However, he had auditory and visual hallucinations. He believed that "little" Japanese army people were coming into his room. He said, "They're very little people. About four of them came to see me today. I'm not afraid of them. They say they are there to help me and that they won't hurt me." During the assessment, there were signs of other delusions as well as tangential and circumstantial thought processes. An extensive evaluation resulted in the diagnosis of schizophrenia, undifferentiated type. His primary care physician prescribed neuroleptic medication with good results.

Reversible dementias include those with a psychiatric cause and metabolic or systemic disorders with symptoms of dementia. Major depression is the most common form of psychopathology with features similar to dementia. Often, there are problems with memory, motivation, concentration, attention, and language. Sleep disturbance is common. As was discussed earlier, schizophrenia can present as dementia. Individuals with anxiety disorders can often have cognitive problems. Dementia syndrome can result from drug toxicity. In the elderly population, use of benzodiazepine, barbiturates, and some of the neuroleptic and antidepressant medications can result in clouded sensorium, confusion, and problems with thought processes. Pharmacological considerations in the treatment and mistreatment of Alzheimer's and other dementias in the elderly is discussed in Chapter 16.

Chronic alcoholism can lead to thiamine deficiency, which is a causal factor of Wernicke–Korsakoff syndrome. These result in impaired expressive language ability.

Nonpsychotropic drugs—including diuretics, cardiac medication, antimonic medication, analgesics, and antihypertension drugs—can impair cognitive abilities. This is especially true with elderly patients where metabolism has slowed, and toxic buildup is more likely to occur than with the general public.

Chemical poisoning can also result in symptoms of dementia, including confusion and delirium. However, these causes of dementia, like the others mentioned, are treatable.

Metabolic disorders that are treatable or reversible include hypoglycemia and hyperglycemia, which often present as delirium. Thyroid disease can result in problems with attention and memory. Dulling of thought processes is associated with hypercalcemia in some instances. Associated features of Cushing's syndrome are depression and delirium. Systemic infection and fever often cause cognitive impairment in the elderly. Pneumonia and urinary tract infections are the most common type. Congestive heart failure and anemia can result in problems with concentration, low energy, and impaired cognition.

Pulmonary diseases often cause delirium. The severity of the problems in such instances tend to increase in the evenings. This is called *sundowning* and is reported often in nursing homes and intensive care facilities. Other reversible dementias include those related to vitamin deficiency, head trauma, neoplasm, hydroencephalus, and multiple sclerosis.

Medical workups are important primarily to identify a reversible form of dementia and treat the cause. In some instances, there may be a form of irreversible dementia that is exacerbated by a medical disorder. Treatment of the medical disorder is then undertaken to diminish the severity of the symptoms of dementia.

The two primary types of irreversible dementia are Alzheimer's and vascular dementia. Other forms of irreversible dementia include dementia due to HIV disease, head trauma, Parkinson's disease, Huntington's disease, Pick's disease, and Creutzfeldt–Jakob disease.

In the diagnosis of vascular dementia, there must be evidence of cerebrovascular disease. Symptoms associated with vascular dementia are usually very specific and focal. Associated features include abnormal reflexes, weakness of an extremity, and gait disturbance. The onset of vascular dementia is usually earlier than with Alzheimer's. Unless there is additional injury, the deficits remain constant. Treatment of hypertension and vascular disease is important in preventing further damage. CT or MRI examinations are often used to detect the extent of the central nervous system lesions. Vascular dementia is usually caused by multiple strokes with the presence of multiple lesions.

Dementia due to HIV disease is characterized by problems with memory, slow thought processes, and problems with problem solving. Often, the individual suffering from the disorder is lethargic, apathetic, and withdrawn. Tremor, anoxia, and repetitive motor activity are associated features. Depression and feelings of hopelessness have also been reported. Central nervous system tumors and dementia from related infections may also be present.

The degree and nature of the cognitive impairments as the result of head trauma, of course, depend on the degree and nature of the injury. Amnesia, as well as continuing problems with memory, are common features. Other associated features are aphasia, problems with attention, anxiety, mood lability, and personality change. The dementia is usually not progressive as in Alzheimer's. Also, there must be evidence of the head trauma to support the diagnosis.

Parkinson's disease is a slow, progressive neurological disorder, with tremor, rigidity, and problems with balance as the primary symptoms. Dementia is frequently a related condition, especially in the more elderly patients. Specific cognitive impairments include problems with planning, organization, and memory retrieval. Motor processes tend to slow. Depression is a commonly associated condition.

Huntington's disease is inherited, progressive, and insidious in nature, with onset usually in the late 30s and 40s. Problems with memory, executive functioning, and judgment are early symptoms. Depression, irritability, and anxiety are common. Disorganized speech and psychosis often appear in late-stage Huntington's. These symptoms and the progressive debilitating nature of the disorder are similar to Alzheimer's. However, a medical examination can differentiate between the two disorders. Because 50 percent of the children of individuals with Huntington's develop the disorder, genetic testing with backup counseling is suggested.

Pick's disease is also a degenerative disease of the brain, with frontal and temporal lobe damage most prominent. Personality changes develop early in the course of the disorder, with deterioration in social skills and poor impulse control. Problems in attention, memory, and language follow. The differentiation between Alzheimer's and

Pick's disease is difficult. However, in Pick's disease, personality changes appear to be more radical and occur earlier in the disorder. Problems with impulse control also tend to be more severe and predominant, with inappropriate social behavior common.

Creutzfeldt–Jakob disease is an infectious disease with a rapidly progressive dementia that is irreversible. Death usually occurs from six months to a year after onset. Extrapyramidal signs tend to appear with myoclonia and burst suppression electroencephalogram (EEG) activity common.

CHAPTER 6

Biological Basis of Dementia

Alzheimer's disease is an organic disorder; however, a psychological or neuropsychological assessment and a social/functional evaluation are necessary in addition to a medical history and medical examination. This is because Alzheimer's is also a functional disorder with cognitive, emotional, and behavioral disturbances.

A medical examination can identify physical illnesses which present symptoms similar to Alzheimer's, such as Parkinson's disease and limbic encephalitis; however, a medical evaluation does not evaluate one's emotional state or identify the specific nature and extent of cognitive impairments and disabilities. More information is needed to develop a treatment and management plan once it has been determined that the causal factors related to dementia are not reversible.

CT or MRI can identify structural pathology; however, this provides no information about the nature of the disability. An assessment focusing on cognitive and behavioral deficits such as memory, attention, language, and abstract reasoning is necessary.

An accurate diagnosis and the development of a treatment and management plan require a comprehensive assessment, including medical, pharmacological, cognitive, and behavioral evaluations. Psychodynamic, family interaction issues, and management considerations must be taken into account. The cooperation of various professionals, including the primary care physician, neurologist, psychologist, nurses, social workers, and physical and occupational therapists, is important.

The first step in an assessment is to distinguish between reversible and irrreversible types of dementia. In the case of reversible dementias, the disease or disorder should be treated. The second step of the assessment is to differentiate between Alzheimer's and other forms of irreversible dementia in order to develop a treatment and management plan. This chapter focuses on the medical evaluation of the dementias as well as biological factors. A medical evaluation includes the physical examination, neurological examination, and various laboratory tests. Chapters 14, 18, and 21 discuss neuropsychological testing, pharmacological considerations, and management techniques.

The medical examination usually begins with a medical history to determine the nature and extent of the presenting problem. Consultation with a family member is often justified to provide for reliability. It is important to determine not only the extent of the problems but also such things as onset and progression. An acute onset tends to rule out Alzheimer's disease and to suggest other factors such as a CVA or other form of injury. Patchy dementia is most common among patients who have suffered from multiple TIAs. Deficits are focal and specific. Individuals who suffer from frontal lobe dementia tend to have problems with judgment, with personality changes common. Temporal lobe dementia often results in agnosia and apraxia.

A history should also include questions regarding medications taken and background of previous disorders and illnesses, as well as a family history of illnesses. This history should include psychopathology as well as current and recent psychosocial stressors. Use and abuse of alcohol and other mood-altering drugs should be discussed and exposure to toxins ruled out.

The physical examination should focus on diseases that present as dementia or have similar symptoms. Laboratory tests often used include evaluations of electrolytes, glucose, calcium, and phosphorus levels; liver, renal, and thyroid functioning; tests for syphilis; vitamin deficiency; and concentration of folic acid.

Other specific procedures include computerized tomography (CT), EEG, skull X ray, MRI, and single-proton emission computerized tomography (SPECT). A skull X ray is of little value in the assessment of dementia. An EEG provides information about the overall integrity of the cerebral cortex and gives evidence of specific disorders such as seizure or Creutzfeldt–Jakob disease. An EEG can also provide data regarding the possibility of lesions, strokes, and tumors. Computerized tomography can identify demyelinization, bleeding, and infarction, as well as loss of tissue and atrophy. CT is valuable in the diagnosis of Huntington's and Pick's disease. However, a normal CT scan is not unusual in the case of Alzheimer's. The MRI is expensive and requires the cooperation of the patient, which is often not possible in cases of Alzheimer's. The SPECT measures blood flow in the brain and can be an important differential diagnosis tool related to vascular dementia. However, according to research, there are not specific patterns suggesting Alzheimer's disease. Lumbar puncture is used primarily where an infectious, inflammatory, or immune disease is possible or suspected.

In dementia due to HIV disease, neuropathology is usually diffuse with destruction of the white matter and subcortical structures. The spinal fluid may have elevated levels of protein with a mild lymphocytosis. Dementia is associated with central nervous system infection.

Parkinson's disease results from neuronal loss and Lewy bodies in the substantia nigra. Patients with Huntington's disease present with atrophy of the striatum. Hypometabolism is often present in the early stages of the disease. Pick's disease affects the frontal and temporal lobes primarily, with evidence of atrophy in these areas. Functional brain imaging may also show frontal and temporal lobe hypometabolism. An EEG with periodic sharp activity is usual in Creutzfeldt–Jakob disease.

Various organic abnormalities have been identified with Alzheimer's disease. Initially, Alzheimer's was considered to be "a weakness of old age." However, in the 1970s, studies identified structural pathology with neuritic plaques and neurofibrillary tangles. Recent studies suggest that the proteins ACT and ApoE4 might be related to fibrous clumps seen in Alzheimer's patients. Neurochemical abnormalities were also suggested with a decrease in the enzyme choline acetyltransferase, suggesting a deficit in a specific neurotransmitter. Loss of subcortical neurons was also suggested. Other findings identified genetic factors. A possible autoimmune etiology was also suggested.

While progress is being made to detect soluble antigens in the central nervous system, there are no laboratory tests that can specifically diagnose Alzheimer's. The diagnosis is based on the specific cognitive impairments as discussed in Chapter 2. Signs of brain atrophy may or may not be evident on the CT or MRI scans. A general medical exam will rule out other medical causes of dementia. However, a mental status exam and neuropsychological evaluation are necessary to identify the degree and level of cognitive disturbance.

Just as laboratory tests cannot be used for the diagnosis of Alzheimer's (only ruling out other forms of dementia), there is no cure for Alzheimer's. However, research continues with some progress and hope. Most of the research focuses on treating cholinergic neurotransmitter deficits. More recently, other neurotransmitter deficits have been studied, including the transmitters norepinephrine, serotonin, and somatostatin. Use of cerebral vasodilators, nootropic medications, and psychostimulants has also been considered in treatment of Alzheimer's. These have not been found to provide significant benefits. Cholinergic neural tissue transplants have also been considered. At this time, therapeutic attempts to remediate or reverse the cognitive impairments have not been successful. However, an early and accurate diagnosis and management plan can improve quality of life not only for the Alzheimer's patient but also for significant others.

CHAPTER 7

Summary: The Dementias Affecting the Elderly

DSM-IV defines *dementia* as an organic disorder resulting in cognitive impairments due to physiological conditions and severe enough to disrupt social and functional abilities. Specific impairments can include memory problems, aphasia, apraxia, agnosia, and problems with executive functions.

There are two types of dementia: reversible and irreversible. The reversible dementias can be treated. The irreversible ones cannot. The importance of an accurate and adequate diagnosis is primary in order to differentiate between the two types of dementia. Failure to make an accurate and complete diagnosis and failure to identify the impairments and spared abilities and resources results in mistreatment and mismanagement. The cases in the Prologue and Chapter 1 illustrate the disastrous results from misdiagnosis—especially in the case of a false positive.

A *false positive* where an individual is falsely diagnosed as suffering from dementia (especially Alzheimer's disease) can result in a self-fulfilling prophecy with the individual assuming the symptoms of dementia. Such was the case with Anna (see Prologue). A false positive can also result in family and staff not providing care or remedial services. A false positive of Alzheimer's rather than identifying reversible forms of dementia can result in failure to treat medical problems and causal factors.

A *false negative*, because of an inadequate or inaccurate diagnosis, can also have a negative impact. Not recognizing the symptoms can result in failure to treat the reversible dementias and failure to manage Alzheimer's. In early-stage Alzheimer's, the family can be educated about the disease and learn ways of interacting with the patient, which reduce anxiety and increase the quality of life. An early and accurate diagnosis helps overcome denial and, in the case of the reversible dementias, allows for intervention before the symptoms become severe.

A *true negative* provides relief for both the individual and the family. However, a true negative based on inadequate data does not explain the causal factors related to the dementia and thus does not necessarily alleviate or remediate the problems. Depression, for example, may result in memory problems and poor attention and concentration. A diagnosis that rules out Alzheimer's is incomplete until data are provided regarding the cause of the symptoms presenting as Alzheimer's. Another problem with a true negative diagnosis is that cognitive functioning changes over time. Recent "pop literature" has provided the general public with a little but not enough knowledge. Checklists and "tests" related to Alzheimer's have been published in the media. Attempting to diagnose Alzheimer's in one's self or a family member is similar to attempting to diagnose cancer. This book is written to provide information about the symptoms of dementias (especially Alzheimer's) and valid diagnostic techniques, based on the premise that the dementias are misdiagnosed, mistreated, and mismanaged. The book is not intended to encourage the layperson to make a diagnosis. Recognition of the symptoms is of value in order to get professional help. Recognition of how many diagnoses of Alzheimer's are based on inadequate information is intended to help the patient and family members differentiate between competent and incompetent professional diagnostic help and techniques.

A *true positive* based on inadequate information can also be harmful if information about the type of dementia and details about the impaired and spared abilities are not provided. A diagnosis must include functional ability information and a treatment and management plan. Too often the diagnosis dementia NOS (not otherwise specified) or "senile dementia" is made by those who present themselves as qualified diagnosticians without inquiry into cause or the provision of a treatment or management plan. Although there may be evidence of dementia, this diagnosis is of little value.

Recent statistics indicate that of the suspected cases of dementia, 55 percent are not reversible. A breakdown of these cases is as follows:

22% Alzheimer's
12% Diffuse causes
12% Vascular dementia
 5% Huntington's or Parkinson's disease
 2% Head trauma

2% Creutzfeldt–Jakob disease

Of the suspected cases of dementia, 34 percent were treatable. Subcategories are as follows:

18% Related to psychological causes
9% Nutritional
4% Lesion related
2% Drug toxicity
1% Hydroencephalitus

Of those cases remaining, 8 percent were not dementia and 3 percent were classified as NOS.

Some of the metabolic and systemic disorders which may present dementia-like syndromes include the following:

Anoxia
Anemia
Congestive heart failure
Vitamin deficiencies
Stroke
Head trauma
AIDS (acquired immune deficiency syndrome)
Other infections
Neoplasm
Cerebral vasculitis
Multiple sclerosis
Cushing's syndrome
Hyperthyroidism
Hypothyroidism
Huntington's disease
Parkinson's disease

This list emphasizes the need for a medical history or examination to rule out the fifty-plus physical illnesses which present symptoms similar to Alzheimer's. Basically, if the symptoms presented are motor deficits; problems with gait; disinhibited behavior; clinical depression; patchy or focal neuropathy; awareness of the problems by the patient with anxiety; and intact language, memory learning, and orientation with personality change, a diagnosis other than Alzheimer's is probable. A more complete discussion of particular disorders and symptoms follows.

DIFFERENTIAL DIAGNOSIS

Age-associated memory impairment (AAMI)

   Not dementia

   Memory impairment only

   Increased time for retrieval of information

   No disorientation

   Ability to learn new information

Alzheimer's disease

   Cognitive impairments

      Memory

      Aphasia

      Apraxia

      Agnosia

      Executive functions

   Emotional behavioral changes

      Early stage—anxiety with confusion and awareness of deficits, irrita-
         bility, some depression

      Middle stage—depression tends to change to anger with the possibility
         of acting out

      Late stage—withdrawn, indifferent, vegetative; often becomes mute;
         unable to care for self

   Progressive degeneration

   Age of onset—late 60s to 80s

   Irreversible

   Pathology

      Cerebral atrophy

      Neuronal loss

      Neurofibrillary tangles

      Neuritic plaques

      Chemical pathology—cholinergic deficiency

   Neuroimaging (CT and MRI)—atrophy or normal

Frontal lobe dementia

   Impairments

      Personality disinhibited or apathy

      Aphasia

      Memory, concentration, construct, calculation abilities more intact than
         with Alzheimer's

   Neuroimaging (CT and MRI)—frontal atrophy

Extrapyramidal syndrome

    Huntington's, Parkinson's progressive supranuclear palsy

    Impairments

        Memory

        Mood and personality changes

        Cognitive dilapidation

        Motor deficits

    Organicity

        Caudate nuclei

        Putamen

        Substantia nigra

        Brain stem structures

Focal sign dementia

    Multi-infarct (vascular dementia)

        Multiple sclerosis

        Subdural hematomas

        Posttraumatic encephalopathy

        Neoplasm

    Impairments—very specific and related to the area of insult or injury; onset follows identifiable trauma or insult; acute in nature; possibility of remediation not progressive

    Neuroimaging (CT and MRI)—specific and focal signs

Depression

    Can be acute or chronic. Life-stage factors such as loss of spouse, physical illness, loss of role and goals, and change of living situation are common psychosocial stressors. These may exacerbate chronic depression symptoms.

    Impairments—memory and concentration problems common; anxiety, lack of energy, sleep disturbance associated features.

    Differs from Alzheimer's in that new information can be learned; usually no language disturbance; in testing the limits, improved performance.

    Neuroimaging (CT and MRI)—no structural evidence

Normal pressure hydrocephalus

    Gait disturbance

    Incontinence

    CT and MRI—enlarged ventricles

    Dementia

Creutzfeldt–Jakob disease

    Rapidly progressive with death six to twelve months after onset

Dementia extremely severe

Burst suppression EEG common

AIDS dementia

Symptoms similar to Parkinson's

Problems with attention, concentration, and memory

Language abilities intact

Tendency to become angry and withdrawn

Alcohol-related dementia

History of alcohol abuse

Memory loss—problems with construct and expressive language; personality change common with disinhibited or apathetic behavior; partial recovery with abstinence

Part II discusses specific diagnostic techniques and procedures.

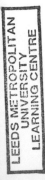

PART II

DIAGNOSTIC TECHNIQUES AND PROCEDURES

CHAPTER 8

Alzheimer's Disease Misdiagnosed: The Mental Status Exam

The advantage of a bad memory is that one enjoys several times the same good things for the first time.

—Nietzsche

The mental status exam is the most commonly used (and misused) instrument to evaluate cognitive abilities such as memory, orientation, attention, concentration, and language function. It is primarily a screening device. When used to diagnose dementia, it can be grossly inaccurate because the test does not provide complete information. The sample of behaviors lacks depth and breadth. False positives are common, with disturbing results, as in the case of Anna (see Prologue). The mental status exam provides only an impression, and a diagnosis based on an impression is not necessarily accurate and valid.

An average or above-average score on the mental status exam tends to rule out dementia, although in the elderly there is some question as to what an average score is. A score of 24 to 30 indicates intact cognitive abilities. A score of 20 to 23 suggests mild impairment; 16 to 19, moderate impairment; and 15 or less, severe impairment. However, these norms do not take into account such factors as physical disability, where motor disabilities may not allow for the completion of such tasks as copying a design or writing a sentence; sensory disabilities, where the subject cannot hear adequately; or problems with orientation due to lack of interest in time and place. This is one of the problems in assessing dementia in the elderly. Many tests and procedures do not have norms for the elderly. The norms for the *Wechsler Adult Intelligence Scale—Revised* (WAIS-R) for example, extend only to age

74. Also, in testing the elderly, there are often sociocultural differences not found in other groups of subjects. For example, problems with language may be related to the fact that English is not the native tongue. More about validity and reliability are presented as the tests used in a neuropsychological evaluation are discussed.

Individuals who do poorly on the mental status exam are not necessarily suffering from dementia. The following two cases illustrate the need for a more complete evaluation.

CASE #14: MICHAEL

The subject is an 87-year-old male who was suffering from arthritis and hip problems. He has a history of CVAs and depression. Family members reported that he was confused, disoriented, and agitated. The family continued that the cognitive deterioration had taken place over a period of about six years, with problems and disabilities becoming more severe. Normally, in the case of vascular dementia, the disabilities follow a CVA or TIA and do not become progressively more severe. However, the cognitive problems could be related to the depression or other medical problems.

The individual scored 11 out of 30 on the mental status exam, suggesting dementia with a provisional diagnosis of Alzheimer's. However, more testing was required to determine the exact nature and extent of the cognitive disability and rule out emotional problems. The comprehensive examination determined that the subject was indeed suffering from severe memory loss (long-term, intermediate, and immediate), aphasia, agnosia, and abstract reasoning. The subject had problems finding words and identifying objects and did not respond to cues. Anxiety did not appear to be a factor in cognitive impairment, and the subject did not display symptoms of major depression. He was not psychotic, although thought processes were severely impaired with inability to make adequate judgments and solve problems. Task completion was impaired because of an inability to follow directions and sequence steps. A diagnosis of dementia of the Alzheimer's type was valid, however, only after a complete evaluation and assessment.

CASE #15: MAY

May was 96 years old and living in a nursing home when assessed. A previous assessment by another examiner had concluded that she was suffering from Alzheimer's. This was based on a brief medical history, a physical examination, and a mental status evaluation. The report indicated that the subject was poorly oriented and had problems with registration, attention, calculation, and language and visual spatial integrity. May scored 24 out of 30 on the mental status exam and scored in the above-average range on the other tests and procedures.

Initially on the reexamination she did poorly. However, this was because of anxiety, lack of interest, and lack of motivation. During the clinical interview, however, rapport was established. She was encouraged to talk about herself and her life. Her mood lifted; and she became more animated, attentive, and invested. During the evaluation, she was encouraged to take her time and relax. Her ability to retrieve information improved. She required a longer time to complete some of the tests than normal; however, this is common with the elderly. As is discussed later, a process approach to evaluation is often more informative than a quantitative approach. With the elderly, testing the limits is important to determine the extent of organicity as well as spared abilities and skills.

The subject had problems identifying the day, date, and year. However, this was not due to organic brain damage; it was due to lack of interest. As she stated, "One day is like the next." Problems in answering questions and following directions, which contributed to a low score on the initial evaluation, were due to a hearing impairment. At first, May denied auditory problems out of pride and lack of interest in the procedure. This illustrates the need for a sensory-perception evaluation as part of a complete assessment. Making sure that the subject heard and understood questions and requests significantly improved results, as did patience, reinforcement, and encouragement. During the assessment, she displayed a good sense of humor, as well as the ability to be interesting, social, and alert. A diagnosis of Alzheimer's had resulted in staff leaving her alone and not encouraging her to become involved socially. She had become isolative, withdrawn, angry, and dysfunctional. Because of a misdiagnosis, she was not being provided the care, attention, and treatment that could have improved the quality of her life. Her abilities were not being used or acknowledged. She was "just another old lady with Alzheimer's"— how sad . . . how tragic.

The mini mental status exam is the most commonly used instrument to diagnosis dementia. As discussed earlier, this instrument should be a screening device only. The administration takes from ten to twenty minutes. If the subject can identify the year, season, date, day, and month, five points are awarded (one point for each correct answer). Elderly individuals, especially those in institutional settings, often do poorly on this task.

The second task is to identify the state; county; town; name of the facility (either where living or tested); and the floor, room number, or home address. Again, one point is given for each correct answer. Elderly individuals often have problems with this task because, in many cases, they have been moved from one living situation to another.

Problems on these two tests can result in the individual losing ten points, which already places them in the mild to moderately impaired category. It might be mentioned that it is not uncommon for the elderly subject to become more confused, anxious, and disturbed when they cannot think of the date or day, thus contributing to additional failures. When the subject is rushed by an impatient examiner, as is often the case where the assessor has many subjects to visit and evaluate in one day, performance problems are exacerbated.

The third task to be completed by the now possibly confused, anxious subject is to repeat three words such as *chair, ball,* and *blue.* One point is given for each correct response. The words or objects can be repeated if the subject fails; however, points are not given. Of course, hearing problems can result in failure.

Five points are given for the famous "serial sevens" test, which requires the individual to subtract 7 from 100 and then continue sequential subtraction. An alternate test is to spell the word *world* forward and backward. While these tasks do not appear to be very complicated, a certain amount of learning is required. Many individuals who are in their 80s and 90s have had little or no formal education. Language problems can also result in poor performance.

The recall task is worth three points if successfully completed. The subject is asked to repeat the three words previously provided (chair, ball, and blue). Elderly individuals often suffer from AAMI and when pushed have problems with retrieval. This does not mean that they are suffering from dementia.

The language tests include naming two objects, such as a pencil and a watch; repeating a statement, such as "no ifs, ands, or buts"; following a three-stage command; writing a sentence; and reading and following a command, such as "close your eyes." Individuals suffering from Alzheimer's, especially during the early stages, tend to maintain some language abilities. Disturbance of language tends to take place in later stages, which often results in the family believing that the individual suffering from Alzheimer's is more able, functional, and capable than is actually the fact. Long-term memory is also maintained more so than intermediate and short-term memory; however, some studies suggest that the extent of retained long-term memory is not as extensive as judged because of the inability to check the accuracy of the information provided by the subject. Individuals suffering from Alzheimer's also often confabulate, especially during the early stages.

The final task on the mini mental status exam requires the individual to copy a design. This is worth one point.

There is a more complete mental status exam; however, it is the opinion of this author that most diagnosticians do not use this form. It is suggested that the most common practice is to briefly interview the family, the patient, or both; review the medical history or perform a brief physical examination; and administer the mini mental status exam or some form of this instrument. It is no wonder that Alzheimer's disease is commonly misdiagnosed, mistreated, and mismanaged.

CHAPTER 9

The Clinical Interview

The clinical interview is one of the richest sources of information regarding a subject's cognitive abilities and emotional state; however, it is often not a part of the diagnostic procedure. The diagnostician tends to review medical records and information and interview the family (usually briefly); but a complete and comprehensive clinical interview is unlikely.

A clinical interview is more than a friendly chat with the subject, although one of the major goals is to put the individual at ease, minimize anxiety, and establish rapport. A clinical interview can be structured or nonstructured. The nonstructured interview is usually more natural and effective in soliciting information in a nonthreatening way. Experience in dealing with people, especially the elderly, tends to lead to an approach that is most comfortable and effective for the individual clinician. Elderly patients are often resistant and somewhat hesitant initially. Beginning the interview with a social remark or commenting on something positive about the person's appearance or dress is usually effective. It is also useful to explain the purpose of the visit or evaluation in simple and honest terms; however, using the word *test* or *assessment* tends to result in some anxiety. I often state that the purpose of the "visit" is to find out "how things are going and if everything is satisfactory." This is especially appropriate in a nursing home. In such a setting, it is also useful to have one of the staff members introduce the examiner to the resident.

Family members can be helpful in preparing the examinee for an evaluation by being honest about their concern and explaining that the examiner is going to help the person with their own concerns and recent problems. As discussed earlier, during the early stages of Alzheimer's disease, there is a tendency to deny problems. Helping the subject improve reality and accept the need for an evaluation will often take tact and require diplomacy. Confrontation is not suggested; however, enumerating recent lapses of memory and other cognitive problems is one approach that often works. It is also important to stress that an evaluation will provide benefits, with a focus on improving functioning and adaptive abilities. Mentioning the possibility of Alzheimer's is not suggested. Family members might, however, share the fact that all of us suffer some problems in memory (i.e., AAMI) and that, as we grow older, retrieval takes more time.

A clinical interview might be started with a sensory-perception examination. This is a useful way to begin once rapport has been established in that the procedure is simple, direct, and nonthreatening. Auditory abilities can be checked by whispering or using a tuning fork. One way of checking vision is to have the subject read words and sentences from the Boston Aphasia Test. The size of print varies. This also allows for the examiner to determine the ability to read and comprehend words and sentences and is a good way to introduce the idea that the subject will be asked to perform various tasks.

During the clinical interview, the diagnostician is encouraged to observe such things as the level of anxiety, the ability to comprehend questions and answer in a logical and appropriate manner, the subject's mood, signs of attention and concentration problems, lack of focus, a tendency to become tangential or circumstantial, symptoms of psychosis, mood swings, signs of regression and decompensation, and the ability to abstract. The way the subject is dressed, manner of speech, body actions and language, and level of mobility should also be observed and notations made. Content, of course, is also important; but just as the process is important in testing, how the subject responds during the clinical interview is important. Information such as resistance to disclose, hesitation in sharing information, disorientation and confusion, problems with cognitive flexibility, negativity, and level of social awareness and appropriateness can be obtained by being alert and observant during the process. Content is important in that it will provide the examiner with information regarding background, family of origin, education, life and job experiences, past trauma and psychosocial stressors, current feelings and emotional state, past and present interests, outlook regarding the future, and family relationships.

While specific information should be solicited, it is often of benefit to allow the subject to proceed at his or her own pace and in his or her own way. Open-ended questions rather than questions which can be answered with "yes" or "no" allow for the subject to express himself or herself more completely and fully. Open-ended questions also allow for the examiner to observe thought processes.

Beginning with one's childhood is a way to establish rapport as well as solicit information. A question such as "What was your childhood like?" is often useful. Asking questions such as "Where did you live?," "How many brothers and sisters did you have?," "What did your father do?," and "What was your parents' marriage like?" allows the examiner to guide the interview and provides the opportunity for the subject to divulge information. Often, such issues as alcoholism in the family, tragedy, or events which occurred during early years and shaped development are disclosed. It is of value to inquire about physical and mental illnesses of the family of origin at this time.

Allowing the subject to discuss adolescent and early adult years provides information on personality characteristics, social and career skills, and adaptive strategies and techniques. Inquiring about interests and hobbies during this period is useful in developing a program to provide the elderly individual with activities and diversions. A man who liked to hunt and fish in his youth can be encouraged to walk and be outdoors. Watching the Discovery Channel on television or getting a subscription to a hunting magazine will allow for the no-longer-active sportsman to have something to look forward to in life. Even in cases where the individual is beginning to show signs of cognitive impairment, there is hope. Looking at pictures with a family member is a possibility.

A woman whose main career and occupation was homemaking may not be able to bake a pie or prepare a meal, but helping to set the table will give the individual a sense of purpose. Folding napkins and sorting silverware are other simple tasks. It is not uncommon in my visits to nursing homes to find individuals with some maintained skills and interests begging to participate in a worthwhile activity.

An extensive clinical interview will not only provide the examiner with information about cognitive functioning but also allow for the formulation of a treatment and management plan based on past interests and maintained abilities.

Exploring the subject's middle adult years often provides information about the sense of self and level of adjustment. How the individual views his or her life experiences and situation is often revealed when discussing this period of life. Unresolved concerns, issues, and problems tend to be discussed and disclosed. How one dealt with trauma and loss in the past helps the examiner estimate how the elderly subject will react in the future.

Discussing recent past events is important in identifying stressors and evaluating emotional state. Old age can be viewed as an opportunity or with great dread and fear. As a part of the clinical interview, I ask the subject about the future. One of my most delightful subjects was a woman who was 101 years old. In response to her view about the future, she took my hand and said, "Honey, this is the future." What a wise remark.

Of course, the information provided during the clinical interview varies with the individual subject. Those who are suffering from late-stage Alzheimer's have limited ability to comprehend questions and express themselves. Individuals who are suffering from psychosis or are agitated, anxious, and resistant present real problems not only in interviewing but also in testing. A calm, patient, understanding approach often breaks barriers and allows for the diagnostician to observe behavior as well as gain information regarding life situation.

In my experience, most of the individuals whom I have tested tend to respond in a positive way to the clinical interview. They enjoy the attention and the opportunity to have someone listen to them. Usually, the experience is therapeutic. However, it must be emphasized that the examiner will be more successful if the process is not rushed. It is not uncommon to spend at least one hour with the subject. This allows the examiner to enter the world of the subject and begin to make judgments not only about cognitive abilities but also about interests, skills, deficits, and emotional state. Without a comprehensive clinical interview, there is the possibility of misdiagnosis, mistreatment, and mismanagement.

CASE #16: MICK THE BULLET

Mick is 92 years old. The clinical interview and assessment took place in a nursing home. Prior to being admitted to the facility, Mick had lived with his second wife, who is 79 years old. One of the reasons that an assessment was ordered was that the wife was requesting power of attorney. She claimed that the subject was unable to care for himself and make reasonable judgments and decisions. The subject had been diagnosed as suffering from dementia of the Alzheimer's type. The staff at the nursing home reported that the resident and his wife had a history of conflict and marital problems.

The subject is a wiry individual with a strong handshake and a slight Irish brogue. He was ambulatory and prided himself on the ability to walk without assistance. During the clinical interview and assessment, he was alert and cooperative. He enjoyed talking about himself and his life.

Visual abilities were intact; however, there were signs of moderate auditory impairment. During the clinical interview it was important to make sure that he could hear and understand questions. Making eye contact and talking loudly and distinctly resulted in improved communication. It was also necessary for the examiner to listen carefully. Too often, especially in cases where there are problems of communication, the receiver does not attend and rushes the interaction. (Refer to Chapter 19.) Some of the interpersonal problems with the wife could be related to poor communication.

During the clinical interview, the subject displayed well-developed language skills as well as intact memories. He had some problems with dates but could recall events from his childhood and adult years. There were no signs of problems with attention or concentration, although he did answer questions in detail. There were signs of narcissistic personality disorder traits and an egocentric focus; however, he was amusing, interesting, and had a good sense of humor.

He stated that he had been born in Ireland and that he had two younger brothers and a sister. His parents came to the United States when he was about 10 years old. He reported that his father worked as a laborer "and drank until he fell down." The father died when he was about 40 years old, and the mother raised the family. The subject reported that while his father was alive, there was marital conflict and abuse. The subject said, "I'm glad my mom and dad fought because it taught me to fight." He continued that at age 17, he began boxing in carnivals and continued to do so until his 30s. He said with pride, "I was called 'Mick the Bullet' because I hit them so fast." The subject admitted that he had a drinking problem much of his life.

He said that he worked as a mechanic and "still likes to repair things." One of the most significant problems in moving to the nursing facility is that he is not able to work in his garage, although he is still physically and mentally able to do so.

The Bullet said that his first wife died about thirty years ago. He described his second marriage as "good." He described the second wife as "one of the finest women who ever walked on two feet on the earth." However, he added that he and the wife had an argument. He continued, "Because of this argument, she put me in here; and I want to go home." He did "go home" soon after this assessment.

The clinical interview was used to provide information not only about cognitive functions but also about life situation factors. The fact that the subject had probably abused alcohol most of his life and suffered many blows to the head alerted the examiner to watch for focal organicity. The clinical interview also provided information related to care and management. Among the recommendations was the suggestion that the husband and wife be seen as a couple to evaluate their relationship and make recommendations regarding their living arrangements.

CHAPTER 10

The Family Interview

An interview with family members or significant others is important in the evaluation of Alzheimer's disease for a number of reasons. History taken over the phone is one way of gathering important data; however, at some time in the procedure, it is beneficial to meet directly with the family as well as interview the family and the subject together. This allows the clinician or diagnostician to evaluate the family system and how the family members interact. These data will be important in making recommendations regarding management and living situations in the future. A family system's approach requires skill and training. It is important for the diagnostician to be able to evaluate blocks in communication, unresolved issues, and the availability of support within the family. Often, there are unresolved issues that result in increased dysfunctional interactions. This may increase the subject's problems. Role reversal is not uncommon, with the parent becoming the child and an adult child family member becoming the caretaker.

Codependency is also not uncommon where the caretaker feels the obligation to provide for needs which might best be met by the subject themselves. Physical illness tends to exacerbate regressive and dysfunctional behaviors. Very often, family members unintentionally make adjustment to intensive care facilities more difficult by being too available. It is not uncommon for a significant other to feel guilt when a family member enters a nursing facility, even when it has been determined that there is a clear and real need for such placement. Being overly attentive or available can result in the patient continuing to be dependent on the family member and not making an effort to stay involved socially and physically. Change is difficult, and there are often many issues of loss and grief connected with aging. The elderly do not always have the ego defenses or adaptive abilities available to younger individuals or available to themselves in earlier times. However, studies have suggested that encouraging the elderly (even Alzheimer's patients) to continue to use spared abilities, both mental and physical, is of benefit. More is presented on the engagement versus disengagement theory and ways of encouraging continued participation and activity later in this chapter.

During the interview with the family member or members, it is also possible to evaluate the level of stress in the family and evaluate expectations and needs. Once these factors are explored, negotiations can be made. Often, the individual who is suffering from Alzheimer's becomes unrealistic and demanding. Irritability, episodes of rage, accusations, suspiciousness, and lack of impulse control result in stress within the family system. Significant others have demands on their time and energies. This is especially true in cases where the elderly parent or parents live in the home of an adult child with a family of their own. A grandmother or grandfather can become the unwanted guest, causing tension and resentment between the generations. This is more common if there has been a personality change, in the cases of acting out, and in situations where physical problems such as incontinence result in time-consuming involvement on the part of the caretaker. The impact of Alzheimer's disease on family members and advice on dealing with these problems is provided in Chapters 22 and 23.

An interview with the family also allows for a more exact evaluation of functional abilities of the subject. Various scales can be used to rate life skill abilities and self-care level. These are discussed in detail in Chapter 15. Of course, the skilled examiner is able—through observation and testing—to make an evaluation about impairments, as well as spared functional capacities. However, in order to develop a management and treatment plan, data regarding at-home abilities are useful. The subject may overestimate and overreport his or her own abilities. He or she may also deny skills as a way of obtaining extra help and attention or eliminating the need to be self-responsible. During the early stages of Alzheimer's, sufferers often confabulate and attempt to hide impairments and problems. Often, maintained language skills result in family members assuming that the individual is more capable than is the case. Family members, especially those closest to the individual with failing capacities, frequently hope for improvement. They look for positive signs. This may be detrimental in the treatment of the Alzheimer's patient because diagnosis is then postponed. Unrealistic hopes and lack of realizing the nature of the disease can result in unrealistic expectations and demands made on the individual with Alzheimer's. This is why an early evaluation is important.

Family members often complain of repetitive questions and what may appear to be volitional carelessness in such things as hygiene. These are symptoms of the disease. There are times and periods where the individual may be more capable than other times. The clinician can best evaluate the level of impairment by getting information from the family, from the patient, and from observation and testing.

An interview with the family member or members is also of educational and therapeutic value. In most cases, it is a relief to talk to a specialist in diagnosing and treating emotional and psychological problems. Family members often are confused and in a state of stress. Common emotional experiences include guilt, anger, frustration, and confusion. The interview with the family allows for some ventilation of these feelings, although short-term family therapy will also be advised to deal with these issues. Once an accurate and valid diagnosis is made, the family can begin to take steps to deal not only with their own feelings but also with the care and treatment of the loved one.

As a part of the evaluation, the family member is asked to bring in the medications currently taken by the subject. This is important in that elderly individuals are often overmedicated. With aging, there are changes in metabolism, with a tendency for toxicity. Also, systemic breakdown can result in drugs staying in the body for a longer time. Psychotropic drugs and mistreatment are discussed in Chapter 17.

A number of instruments are available to the diagnostician in obtaining information. A combination open-end and structured format is suggested. A structured interview allows one to collect specific information in an orderly way. The open-end portion of the interview allows the diagnostician to evaluate the psychodynamics and more subtle elements of the interaction, communication patterns, and family system.

The structured portion of the interview elicits information related to living skills, as well as family impressions regarding cognitive status. It is important to inquire about observed changes in abilities, skills, behavior, and attitude. This is related to the fact that Alzheimer's is a progressive disease. Family members should also be asked to provide a medical history. This history should be checked against medical records (when available, such as in a hospital or nursing home evaluation situation) and the subject's self-report.

Structured questionnaires should cover reports of memory; expressive and receptive language; daily functioning, regardless of whether the individual recognizes the problems; psychiatric, medical, and use-of-alcohol problems; family of origin history related to physical and mental problems; medications; and medical contacts. A consultation with the subject's physician might be of benefit, especially if the primary care physician has been involved in an evaluation for cognitive and functional problems. As discussed earlier, a medical examination might also be warranted.

In the case of a patient who is institutionalized, the staff should also be interviewed. Staff impressions about the nature of the problems and the course are very valuable. Staff are often able to describe interpersonal social abilities, characterological traits, and family support availability and dynamics. All this information is important in making the diagnostic judgments and preparing a management and treatment plan.

Chapters 11 to 15 discuss neuropsychological testing, specific tests and techniques, reliability and validity, and specific problems in testing the elderly. The focus of this discussion is on the dementias.

CHAPTER 11

Special Considerations in the Diagnosis of Alzheimer's

Physicians usually rely on "impressionistic" data to assess Alzheimer's disease in the elderly. As discussed in Chapter 8, a diagnosis is often based on a cursory medical exam and the administration of the mini mental status exam. Usually, this is not sufficient and, in the case of Anna (see Prologue) and thousands of other misdiagnosed Alzheimer's patients, results in severe mental anguish, inadequate treatment of the real disorder, and mismanagement. Too often, the diagnosis of this degenerative, progressively devastating disease is completed by an unqualified assessor using incomplete techniques and tools.

In order for the evaluation to be accurate, the following questions must be answered:

1. Do the symptoms exist as detailed in *DSM-IV*?
2. What are the causal factors of the symptoms?
3. Are these causes treatable and are the symptoms reversible?
4. What abilities and skills are impaired, and what abilities and skills are spared?
5. What is the nature and the extent of the disabilities, and how do they affect cognition and functioning?
6. What are the possibilities for remediation and compensation?

Based on this information, a treatment and management plan can be developed. Failure to complete an accurate assessment, answering all of the above questions and then not developing a treatment plan, is like telling individuals that they have cancer and then abandoning them. In fact, it may be psychologically more damaging. The general public has been educated that cancer is often treatable. Alzheimer's is not, and the public realizes this. It is the moral, ethical, and probably legal obligation of the diagnostician to provide a complete and accurate diagnosis.

An article in the November 11, 1994, *Chicago Sun Times* points out the dangers of an incomplete or inaccurate diagnosis of Alzheimer's. The article, which is titled "New Alzheimer's Test Shows Promise," reports on a test using eyedrops. Harvard University researchers claim that "probable" Alzheimer's patients have pupils that dilate more fully and more rapidly to eyedrops than those who do not have Alzheimer's. The article points out that three other earlier biophysiological tests have not lived up to expectations in diagnosing Alzheimer's and that Harvard researchers admit that the sample size of 100 is small.

The article continues that "a quick diagnosis" of Alzheimer's which may be inaccurate can have "devastating" results and that a wrong diagnosis can be "disastrous." The writer continues to say that using a medical history and neuropsychological test results prove to be 90 percent accurate. Chapter 14 is devoted to the use of neuropsychological tests in the assessment of Alzheimer's. This chapter focuses on issues of reliability and validity in testing the elderly, competency of the assessor, and specific problems in testing the elderly.

Psychology is defined as the scientific observation of human behavior. Neuropsychology is related to making brain behavior observations. More is said about this in Chapter 12. In order for medical as well as psychological and neuropsychological results to be of value, certain principles must be adhered to in the process.

The first principle is related to the competency of the person doing an evaluation. Under law, there are certain procedures that a physician, a psychologist, and a social worker can perform. These professionals are certified, which is related to the use of a title such as "doctor of medicine" or "psychologist," as well as licensed. Licensing refers to the allowable practices and procedures. The terms *counselor* and *therapist* are not licensed and can be used by individuals without any specific training. Licensing law prescribes the type of training and experience necessary in order to practice. Unfortunately, many individuals who are not licensed or certified present themselves as qualified and competent. Chapters 23, 24, and 25 discuss how the family members can find competent help and which questions to ask when arranging for an evaluation for Alzheimer's disease.

As discussed previously, a complete assessment probably should utilize the skills of a physician, a psychologist, and a social worker. A medical doctor is trained to treat medical illnesses. Ruling out a medical illness is important when assessing dementia. The general practitioner is licensed to prescribe medication, including antianxiety medications and other psychotropic drugs. However, they usually do not perform psychological or neuropsychological assessments or treat mental illness. Neurologists diagnose and treat illnesses with a biological or organic basis.

Psychologists, on the other hand, are specialists in observing and assessing human behavior, such as motor abilities and cognitive functions. To repeat, the diagnosis, treatment, and management of dementias require knowledge about such things as memory, language skills, attention, and thinking.

Social workers initially were trained to provide social services to families and individuals. These abilities are invaluable in locating community resources and helping in the management stage. They also can provide social histories. More recently, social workers have entered the field of psychotherapy. However, they cannot, according to licensing law, perform psychological and neuropsychological assessments.

The specifics of a neuropsychological evaluation are discussed in Chapter 14. A few remarks pertaining to the general principles of making an assessment, however, are appropriate. A scientific assessment is more than a casual observation. A psychological test is an objective measure of a sample of behavior. From this sample, predictions are made in regards to a broader area of behavior. In order for this prediction to be accurate, the sample must be large enough for a hypothesis or generalization to be made. This is why the mental status exam has been criticized as a predictor of such cognitive abilities as memory, attention, and language functions and why this book supports a more complete and accurate battery of tests. Asking the individual to provide information about the date or perform serial sevens does not provide sufficient information to diagnose orientation and calculation abilities any more than asking the individual to provide the name of the President of the United States tests fund of knowledge and long-term memory. Identifying two objects like a pen and a watch is inadequate and an insufficient way to diagnose agnosia. Asking the individual to complete a simple three-step task does not test executive functions. There is much more to testing.

A second requirement of scientific observation, in addition to drawing a sufficient and representative sample, has to do with establishing norms. The administration, scoring, and interpretation of the tests should be objective. One of the problems in testing the elderly is that "normal" or average behavioral standards have not been developed. In other words, the person testing an individual for memory abilities may use two or three different tests. However, these data are not of value if there is no way to tell if the performance is in the average range or above or below average. More is said in Chapters 13 and 14 about the lack of norms in testing the elderly, especially in relation to individual differences among same-age cohorts.

Another consideration in testing is reliability, that is, consistency of scores when the same test or an equivalent form of the test is given to the same person. The elderly tend to be influenced by the examiner. An individual who rushes the elderly patient and does not take time to establish rapport often ends up with poor test results. A final consideration is validity. This is related to the degree to which a test actually measures what it purports to measure. As discussed earlier, failure to draw a large enough or representative sample results in confounded data or results.

Testing conditions also affect results. Lighting is an important consideration, as is performing the assessment in an area where there is a minimum amount of distraction and external stimulation. Sufficient time must be allowed so that the subject is not rushed. In testing cognitive and functional abilities, it is allowed to "test the limits." This is different from psychological testing, where encouragement and reinforcement are not allowed. In neuropsychological testing, the examiner is interested in determining the highest level of performance or functioning under optimum conditions.

Prior to the assessment, materials should be arranged. Elderly patients tend to become anxious and distracted when the examiner sets up equipment such as desks and chairs while they are waiting to be tested. When an examiner is well organized and proceeds in a smooth manner, subject anxiety is reduced.

The assessor should also review the medical chart, if available; interview staff; and talk to family in an initial assessment. This is to gather information, not make diagnostic decisions. As discussed earlier, the diagnostic decision is the result of data gathered in a number of different ways and from a number of different sources.

Sensory-perception deficits should be corrected if possible so that these disabilities do not impair performance. In the case of an individual who needs glasses to read, the glasses should be brought to the assessment. The same is true of dentures and hearing aids. Often, speech is difficult to understand because of failure to wear dentures. In the case where dentures are used but not brought to the evaluation, the subject often becomes self-conscious and resists talking to the examiner. Providing for the correction of disabilities not only shows courtesy but also improves performance. If an individual is hearing impaired but can use sign language, an intermediary should be present. The same is true with an individual who does not speak the examiner's language. Better yet, a bilingual examiner might be used. Special editions of some of the tests presented in Chapters 12 and 13 are available for the visual and hearing impaired and those with orthopedic handicaps.

Often, the examiner is required to improvise. In testing the limits to determine whether there is any ability to respond (e.g., with a mute patient), such things as tracking, startle-response tests, tactile stimulation, singing, counting, and repeating the individual's name are used, just as repetition, cuing, pantomime, and demonstration can be used in communicating with middle- to late-stage Alzheimer's patients.

Some suggestions have been made on establishing rapport. The establishment of rapport is very important when testing the elderly, as is reducing anxiety. Starting the assessment procedure before the subject is comfortable and at ease will result in poor performance. Tests tend to threaten one's dignity, sense of self, and prestige. It should be explained that no one is expected "to get all the answers correct" or complete all the tasks perfectly. Reinforcement during the assessment helps keep the individual interested, motivated, and nonthreatened.

The examiner should allow time-outs in situations where anxiety is evident or extreme. Breaking the procedure down into sessions is often necessary when testing the elderly. Also, it might be necessary to limit the number of tests given or to shorten the subtests.

In testing the elderly, it must be realized that recall and retrieval may take a longer time than with younger subjects. Also, considerations must be made regarding level of education, cultural–social factors, and background factors that might confound test results and interpretations. An individual who does not speak the language well or has had no formal education may appear to have Alzheimer's symptoms. Lack of familiarity with specific objects may present as agnosia. Poor performance on tests that measure abstract thinking might be related to cultural factors. Emotional problems such as depression can result in lethargy and disinterest. All of these factors must be considered in testing and in determining the level of cognitive skill and ability. A ten-minute examination is not enough.

CHAPTER 12

The Psychological Assessment

Just as it takes special knowledge and training for the physician to diagnose and treat physical illnesses, it takes special knowledge and training to diagnose cognitive and emotional problems not only in the general public but especially in the elderly. Special test and evaluation techniques and measurements have been developed over time to evaluate emotional problems and mental abilities. These tests and instruments are used to quantify as well as qualify skills and abilities and impairments and disabilities. Individuals who have not had training and supervision are not, under licensing law, allowed to use these instruments.

It has been estimated that 18 percent of the individuals who have been diagnosed as suffering from Alzheimer's disease actually suffer from an emotional disorder or disorders that can be treated. This illustrates the great danger of failing to consider possible causes of dementia other than organic causes. It is important to be aware of the patient's physical problems in order to rule out reversible causes of dementia. This is the purpose of a medical examination. However, Alzheimer's disease cannot be diagnosed on the basis of a brief interview with the patient or family and a medical examination. Psychological and emotional factors must also be assessed. Family members are cautioned to be wary of a diagnosis based only on a medical examination and the use of the mental status exam. Before arrangements are made for an evaluation for Alzheimer's, it behooves the family to inquire about the extent and the nature of the assessment, the procedures used, and the qualifications of the examiner. An individual who is not specifically trained to diagnose physical illnesses should not be allowed to attempt such a task any more than someone who is not trained and does not have specific knowledge should attempt to diagnose emotional, intellectual, and psychological impairments and disabilities.

This is especially important in the diagnosis of Alzheimer's in that the symptoms are primarily cognitive. X ray, CT, and MRI cannot determine language skills, memory functions and attention, orientation, and incidental learning skills any more than can a ten-minute mental status examination.

The first part of this chapter discusses evaluation procedures and instruments commonly used to assess emotional and psychological factors. There is also a brief discussion of limitations in using these instruments and techniques with the elderly, especially where cognitive or physical abilities are impaired.

Chapters 13 to 15 discuss intellectual and neuropsychological testing. Part II concludes with a summary of suggested tests and procedures to be used in a complete assessment battery.

It has been estimated that from 7 to 10 percent of the population suffers from major depression. This percentage appears to be higher among the elderly. This is probably due to life situation factors that exacerbate symptoms of depression. Changes in lifestyle and life situation cause stress. Inability to deal with stress tends to result in physical and emotional illness. People who have jobs, families, and other support systems are more able to cope with psychosocial stressors and physical illness. The elderly, in many cases, have lost support systems and are more vulnerable to stress. The physical aging process and the loss of the ability to function independently causes frustration and dysphoria. Loss of loved ones, roles, and an active and productive life add to depression, often with feelings of hopelessness and uselessness.

The elderly also tend to suffer from anxiety because of concerns about their future health and security. Depression and anxiety can present as dementia. It has been the experience of this examiner that many of the individuals who have been diagnosed as suffering from Alzheimer's in fact suffer from major depression and/or generalized anxiety disorder.

Psychological tests are used to measure differences between individuals or between how one individual responds in different situations or occasions. Some of the problems associated with assessing emotional states in the elderly have been presented. Two specific tests for depression are discussed here, with a focus on limitations and uses.

The first test, which is commonly used to evaluate for depression, is *The Beck Depression Inventory* (BDI), developed by Aaron T. Beck and Robert A. Steer in 1987. The test, along with other psychological tests, is not available to the general public. This is because of the need for special training and supervision in the administration and interpretation of the results. Psychological diagnosis is based on the formulation of various hypotheses and then the acceptance or rejection of these hypotheses based on data. These data must be valid (i.e., test or measure what is supposed to be tested) and reliable. Validity and reliability are discussed in Chapter 11. A diagnosis of depression, for example, must be based on data from various sources, such as behavioral observation, a clinical interview, and various objective (and possibly subjective) tests. Just as Alzheimer's disease cannot be diagnosed from the administration of the mental status exam, major depression cannot be diagnosed by data provided from one test such as the BDI, although this test and others discussed do provide general guidelines and cut off scores for various levels of depression.

A word about these guidelines or "norms" is appropriate at this time. Norms are based on the performance of a sample of the general population. The sample size must be large enough to be representative of the total population. Samples are often taken from various age groups or sociocultural groups in an attempt for the norms to be representative. The smaller the sample size, the less likely it is to be representative. However, it is impossible from a practical basis to draw a very large sample because of cost considerations.

One problem in using quantitative tests with the elderly is that many tests do not have norms for elderly individuals. The scales on the WAIS-R run from ages 16 to 74. Many of the individuals tested for Alzheimer's are more than 74 years of age. Another problem in using tests is that elderly individuals often are unable to complete the tests for various reasons. This is true, especially for some of the self-report personality tests, which require the subject to answer from 150 to over 400 questions. This is tedious and often difficult for younger individuals. Fatigue and lack of interest and motivation factors can become very significant.

The BDI consists of twenty-one groups of four statements. The statements reflect symptoms and attitudes associated with depression, including mood, pessimism, sense of failure, self-dissatisfaction, guilt, punishment, self-dislike, self-accusation, suicidal ideation, crying, irritability, social involvement, indecisiveness, body image, work problems, insomnia, fatigue, loss of appetite and weight, somatic concern, and libido. The original version of this inventory was to be read to the subject (which is often necessary with elderly subjects) rather than having the subject read and choose the response that applies to them personally. This test takes from ten to fifteen minutes to administer to the average subject but may take much longer in the case of an elderly patient. Partial administration focusing on sadness, pessimism, guilt, suicidal ideation, self-dislike, and withdrawal may be necessary and of benefit to the diagnostician. However, this does not provide a score which can be quantified. This does provide data for further investigation of mood. The data provided can be used to develop a treatment and management plan. Asking the subject whether they are "depressed," as is commonly done during a medical examination, is insufficient.

Another instrument which can be used to gather information about mood is the *Beck Hopelessness Scale* (BHS), originated by Aaron T. Beck (1988). This test consists of twenty statements regarding attitudes about the future. The test has been used to predict suicidal intentions. The test can be self-administered or administered orally. Again, norms are provided but not for the elderly specifically. Both of these tests require that the subject comprehends the questions.

Self-report inventories such as the *Minnesota Multiphasic Personality Inventory* (MMPI) are instruments for the measurement of emotional, motivational, interpersonal, and attitudinal characteristics. The MMPI consists of 550 affirmative statements to which the subject responds true or false. Items on the test cover such areas as health, psychological and neurological disorders, symptoms, motor disturbance, social attitude, and marital issues. Ten clinical scales are provided from the data obtained on the MMPI, three of which are depression, hysteria, and schizophrenia.

Other self-report inventories with fewer questions are also available to identify symptoms of emotional disorder. However, because of time and cost limitations when assessing Alzheimer's, self-report inventories are not often used.

Projective techniques are instruments that are subjective rather than objective, although interpretive guidelines and norms have been developed. A projective test requires the subject to perform a relatively unstructured task such as making up a story when presented with a picture. A test such as this might be of some value in providing information about the subject's emotional state in that the content and the theme of the story reflect the subject's view of self and the world. The story itself and how it is told can provide data about thought processes and abstract ability. Other tests that have been used to diagnose depression, anxiety, and schizophrenia include the sentence-completion test and sentence-writing tests. The first test requires the subject to complete a sentence stream such as "I become sad when . . ." or "I become angry when. . . ." Of course, in order to complete the sentence, a certain amount of comprehensive ability is required, which many Alzheimer's patients do not possess. Content of the completed statements (which can be read to the subject) provides data on his or her mood. Another technique involves asking the respondent to write a sentence of his or her own. This also provides insight regarding mood and preoccupation.

These are only a few of the tests and instruments used to diagnose mood. The abilities and nonimpaired cognitive functions of the patient suspected of Alzheimer's, of course, determine the tests that are appropriate. During early-stage Alzheimer's, it is more possible to assess mood disorders that may be coexisting with dementia. As the disease progresses, the dementia becomes primary. Chapters 13 and 14 discuss intellectual and neuropsychological testing procedures and techniques. These also provide information about the possibility of depression, anxiety, and schizophrenia, which is helpful to the diagnostician. In some cases, signs of mood or thought disorder are obvious, such as in the case of hallucinations or psychotic thoughts when asked to complete a task. In other cases, symptoms are less obvious, such as lack of motivation, low energy, and lack of interest, suggesting depression.

The trained and competent diagnostician has many techniques and procedures to utilize in differentiating mood disorders from Alzheimer's. The purpose of this chapter was to discuss a few and emphasize the need for a complete and thorough assessment. The family of an individual who has been assessed, after a cursory examination, as suffering from Alzheimer's should insist on a second opinion by a competent and qualified examiner.

CHAPTER 13

Assessing Intellectual Abilities

The *Wechsler Adult Intelligence Scale—Revised* (Wechsler 1981) is one of the most widely used tests in psychological assessment and recently was revised as a neuropsychological instrument. The WAIS-R measures mental abilities but also provides data on emotional and characterological factors. Scores on the eleven subtests can be used to discover how the individual subject ranks related to average ability. Because the test measures cognitive ability, both verbal and nonverbal, it is an essential tool in the assessment of disorders such as dementia. As discussed in Chapter 2, symptoms of Alzheimer's include problems with memory, planning and organizing, attention, orientation, and language.

The first subtest (Information) is a test of fund of knowledge and an indicator of long-term memory and orientation. A low score on this test suggests that the respondent is unable to retrieve information such as how many days there are in a week. (The mental status examination provides some data on memory but is not as effective or efficient in measuring the level of ability.) One of the factors that should be considered in administrating this test is the possibility of respondent anxiety. This is especially true in testing the elderly. The subject might be cautioned not to become disturbed if they do not know all the answers. Scaled scores have been provided for individuals of various ages, including those between 70 and 74; however, there are no scale age equivalent scores above this. With an aging population, norms for those above age 74 should be developed.

The second verbal subtest (Digit Span) requires the individual to repeat digits both forward and backward. Forward digits are given first. The number of digits increases from 2 to 9 in digits forward and 2 to 8 in digits backward. This test is for immediate auditory memory.

The task also requires the individual to attend and concentrate. Digits backward is more difficult in that it requires reverse sequencing. Individuals with Alzheimer's perform poorly on both parts of this test. Often, they are unable to repeat even two digits backward. In cases of middle-stage dementia, it is necessary, in many cases, to repeat the directions a number of times as well as demonstrate. Of course, abilities vary with individuals and many elderly individuals are able to perform digits forward and backward. In one testing situation, a 97-year-old woman was able to perform digits forward. However, when asked to repeat the digits backward, she stated, with a smile on her face, "I can't do that; I'm 97 years old." When given encouragement, however, she scored in the above-average range.

Individuals who have left hemisphere brain damage tend to have problems with both parts of the test. There have been some reports that right frontal lobe damage impairs digits backward performance more so than digits forward. Anxiety states affect performance on digits forward and backward; however, results are fairly normal for schizophrenics without cognitive deterioration.

The third verbal subtest (Vocabulary) has been recognized as the best single indicator of intelligence; however, results can be affected by level of education, knowledge of the English language, and cultural factors. Many individuals in their 80s are not native Americans, and English is not their primary tongue. In one case of testing, an 82-year-old Hispanic woman did well on this test initially but, as the words became more difficult, regressed and began to think in Spanish.

In Alzheimer's disease, there tend to be problems with both receptive and expressive language. The WAIS-R Vocabulary test measures expressive language in that the individual is required to define words. The Boston Aphasia and Boston Naming tests, which are discussed in Chapter 14, are neuropsychological tests that are more specific and test for aphasia and agnosia.

In most cases, the Vocabulary test gives an indication of premorbid ability in that vocabulary is one of the last areas of deterioration in situations of brain damage. This does not apply in cases of Alzheimer's where language abilities tend to deteriorate in early to middle stages. At times, however, the individual does maintain the ability to converse with family members on a very concrete level. Long-term memory functions, when compared to intermediate and immediate memory functions, are also maintained at times. Unfortunately, this often gives the family members the impression that the individual is more capable and functional. However, thought processes are usually very concrete with problems in abstraction and assimilation of new information.

The Arithmetic subtest requires the respondent to solve word problems. This test is very important in that it indicates the individual's ability to solve daily problems in logic. A certain amount of arithmetic knowledge is required; however, the test begins with very simple problems. This test also measures verbal understanding, memory, and concentration. Impairments in these areas are symptoms of Alzheimer's. In testing the elderly, there is often resistance to this subtest with the assertion by the individual that they are unable to perform the test just as the 97-year-old woman jokingly resisted digits backward. The Arithmetic test, as well as the performance on the Digit Span test, is a good indicator of anxiety. Individuals with left hemisphere brain damage tend to do poorly on this test.

The Comprehension test measures the individual's knowledge of social norms and expectations. This test is a good indicator of long-term memory and the ability of the individual to verbalize. Individuals suffering from depression or anxiety are more able to perform on this test than those with Alzheimer's. Cognitive abilities tend to be intact in individuals with emotional problems, whereas Alzheimer's patients lose sense of propriety and social custom. This is one reason they tend to act in inappropriate ways as the disease progresses. Impulse control is also diminished. Individuals who are suffering from schizophrenia often give bizarre or odd responses. Good scores on the Comprehension test suggest that the person is oriented.

The final verbal subtest is Similarities. This test measures abstract reasoning and the ability to form verbal concepts. The test requires memory, concentration, language ability (both receptive and expressive), and the ability to attend. Individuals with Alzheimer's tend to do poorly on this test. An average or above-average score on the Similarities test suggests good verbal planning and organization skills with the ability to generalize. One of the major problems facing individuals with Alzheimer's is that they cannot assimilate information. This is due, in part, to memory impairment. Inability to learn new information makes adaptation to new situations difficult.

There are five WAIS-R nonverbal tests that require visual, spatial, and motor skills. Just as performance on the verbal tests may be impaired by auditory problems and speech disabilities, problems may arise on the nonverbal WAIS-R tests because of paralysis, fine motor problems, and visual problems. The examiner should allow for such impairments and disabilities.

The visual–spatial motor subtests are called Performance tests. Because Alzheimer's disease is a disease that impairs primarily verbal abilities, the examiner may use only a few of the nonverbal tests. This does not allow for the determination of a full scale score; however, this is not as significant as it may be in assessments of other populations. The examiner may also limit the number of verbal tests. This is dependent on such factors as time available, cooperation of the respondent, and the respondent's capacity for testing. In cases of middle- to late-stage Alzheimer's, the WAIS-R may be used as a screening device or specific tests used to test particular areas of cognition. This applies to the tests mentioned in Chapter 14. While it would be of benefit to use all of the tests suggested, in some cases, it is often not practical.

The first performance test is the Picture Completion subtest. The respondent is asked to identify an essential detail that is missing in a picture. This is a test of visual organization and perception and requires attention to detail. Schizophrenic patients tend to identify odd or bizarre parts. Individuals who are depressed tend to give up easily and do not persist. Patients with Alzheimer's often do not understand the task at hand.

The second test is Picture Arrangement, where the individual is asked to place a number of cards with pictures on them in the proper sequence. In some ways, this is similar to the Comprehension test in that the respondent must have a knowledge of social norms and appropriate behaviors. This test also measures executive functions, which are impaired in individuals with Alzheimer's. Cognitive reasoning and flexibility are also tested. One problem with this test is that there may be a cultural bias. This should be considered in the evaluation. Individuals with vascular dementia do not necessarily do poorly on this test unless the brain damage is in the right frontal area. Some left hemisphere injuries may also impair social knowledge and skill. Individuals with Alzheimer's tend to have significant problems with this test, as do psychotic patients. Depressed and anxious patients tend to maintain social knowledge, both verbal and nonverbal.

The third performance test is Block Design. The subject is asked to place blocks in such a way as to duplicate a design on a card. This is the best indicator of nonverbal reasoning and is often used in assessing brain injuries involving either the right or left parietal lobe. Schizophrenics tend to score at or above the mean score. The low score for the brain-damaged individual differentiates organicity from psychosis. Anxious or impulsive individuals have problems with this subtest—as do Alzheimer's patients—because of problems with organization and planning.

The Object Assembly test requires visual analysis and visual motor skills. In this test, the subject is required to assemble a puzzle. Recognizing interrelationships of parts is important. Individuals suffering from Alzheimer's, organic brain damage, and schizophrenia tend to do poorly on this test, as do depressed individuals. Because of this, the Object Assembly test does not provide much data on a differential diagnosis.

The last nonverbal test is the Digit Symbol test. This test requires intact motor skills. The individual is asked to place symbols below numbers. Each number has its own symbol. This test measures non-verbal memory and learning. In order to do well, the respondent must memorize the digit number relationship. Individuals with Alzheimer's cannot do this because incidental learning and memory (both visual and auditory) tend to be impaired. Because this is a timed test (as are a number of other tests), individuals suffering from anxiety do poorly. Depressed individuals tend to go slowly.

The preceding description of the WAIS-R illustrates how a test such as this not only provides extensive information about impaired versus spared abilities but also can be used to differentiate between the various emotional disorders and dementias. It is important to emphasize that these tests must be administered, scored, and interpreted by a trained and knowledgeable examiner and that a diagnosis should not be made on the basis of limited data.

The WAIS-R test provides a great deal of information regarding cognitive problems and possible causes. The WAIS-R has been used in the past as a neuropsychological instrument. In 1991, a new edition was issued. This is called WAIS-R-NI or the *Wechsler Adult Intelligence Scale—Revised—Neuropsychological Instrument*. The reason for this new edition is based on the assertion that the WAIS-R limits information because a raw score is provided with little information on the particular type of deficits. For example, a respondent is not given credit for four out of five cards arranged correctly on the Picture Arrangement test any more than a subject is given credit if none of the cards are in order.

Kaplan, Fein, Morris, and Delis emphasize the importance of observing the process rather than focusing strictly on the content or the quantitative factors. The WAIS-R-NI is designed to answer the needs of both the clinical psychologist and the neuropsychologist by providing a way to analyze the various aspects of the process. Testing the limits is important in neuropsychology in that it allows the clinician to identify spared and maintained abilities that might be the focus of remediation or therapy. Reinforcing the subject is important, just as is the elimination of stress and anxiety if possible. Additional neuropsychological tests and concepts are discussed in Chapter 14.

CHAPTER 14

Neuropsychological Testing
for Dementia

The WAIS-R, especially when used as a neuropsychological instrument, is a very sophisticated and effective tool for evaluating organic brain damage. The WAIS-R is used in research and treatment facilities that focus on brain damage and injury and treatment and remediation.

Alzheimer's disease is an organic brain disease; however, too often the diagnosis is performed by individuals with little training or background in the assessment of organicity. Anna (see Prologue) is an example of the danger of misdiagnosis of Alzheimer's. Until an individual with the symptoms of Alzheimer's is properly diagnosed by a trained and qualified diagnostician with knowledge of brain behavior relationships, there continues to be the risk of misdiagnosis, mistreatment, and mismanagement.

In previous chapters, we have discussed some of the procedures for gathering data for a valid diagnosis. This chapter focuses on the neuropsychological assessment and the use of various neuropsychological tests and techniques related to Alzheimer's disease.

A neuropsychological assessment is concerned with the diagnosis of brain damage or organicity. Interest in developing noninvasive methods to test for organicity began in the 1930s. The Halstead–Reitan Neuropsychological Test Battery was one of the first instruments and was the result of work by Ward Halstead at The University of Chicago. Halstead's research was with brain-damaged individuals. Halstead's work was continued by Ralph Reitan, who established a neuropsychological laboratory at The University of Chicago. Eventually, a battery was developed to measure a broad range of abilities.

The purpose of a neuropsychological evaluation is to aid in diagnosis, establish a baseline for future performance, estimate the prognosis, and develop a treatment plan. Dementias in the elderly have various causes. Some of them are reversible. Because of this, it is important to differentiate between Alzheimer's and systemic or functional dementias that can be treated. It is also important to identify the level and extent of impairment and which skills and abilities have been spared. Neuropsychological assessment techniques allow the trained diagnostician to make an accurate diagnosis and predictions. A neuropsychological evaluation in the assessment of dementia focuses primarily on cognitive abilities. Identifying cognitive deficits among those with middle- or late-stage Alzheimer's disease is often rather easy. However, early-stage Alzheimer's is more difficult to diagnose; and many of the symptoms of other forms of dementia are very similar.

This chapter focuses on specific tests as well as general approaches. The WAIS-R provides data on mental abilities or intelligence but does not always predict functional ability. As discussed previously, a low score on the WAIS-R could be related to depression, anxiety, or situational factors. A neuropsychological evaluation provides more specific data in such areas as visual–spatial motor skills, the ability to abstract, memory, agnosia, and aphasia. This does not mean that every patient suspected of suffering from Alzheimer's disease should or can be given a complete neuropsychological evaluation. However, various tests and assessment techniques can be used by the neuropsychologist to differentiate between types of expressive language problems and causes, for example, or to assess deficits in attention and concentration and make an appraisal of causal factors.

A neuropsychological assessment can also provide data on chronicity of the symptoms and prognosis for continued deterioration. Comparing current performance with past performance and considering level of education, occupation, and previous functional abilities allow the diagnostician to estimate the severity of the impairments and make predictions about the future. Poor performance by an individual with limited premorbid abilities does not necessarily indicate dementia. It is important to distinguish between mental retardation and dementia.

A neuropsychological assessment is often of benefit to evaluate the level of impairment when reports of the family and the report of the individual differ. The assessment is also of value in medical situations where the results of a procedure can be evaluated. In the case of vascular dementia, cognitive abilities may improve with time. An assessment can also be of benefit in measuring response to various medications. Chapter 17 discusses the use of psychotropic medications with the elderly. Some of these medications have side effects, which can increase confusion, cause anxiety and excitement, and increase risk of falling.

Initially, test batteries were used in an attempt to differentiate between patients who were suffering from brain damage and those who were not.

The rationale was that this differentiation could be made based on an accumulation of failures in various areas of cognitive functioning, both verbal and nonverbal. There was also increased emphasis on lateralization and localization of brain lesions. The Halstead–Reitan Neurological Test Battery and the Luria–Nebraska Neuropsychological Battery were and still are the primary instruments used for this purpose. Proponents of these test batteries report that these instruments can detect and lateralize lesions more accurately than with the use of CT. This may or may not be; however, these batteries are usually not given in their entirety in the diagnosis of Alzheimer's. One reason is that Alzheimer's presents primarily and initially with very specific cognitive symptoms. In review, these are memory impairment, aphasia, apraxia, agnosia, and disturbance in executive functions. Testing verbal abilities is primary, although the diagnostician can test such functions as nonverbal memory and visual–spatial motor skills by using the Bender–Gestalt direct-copy, immediate recall, and delayed recall tests.

Using specific tests to evaluate such functions as memory; the ability to name objects; language impairments; and the ability to plan, attend, and organize has become more common in evaluating dementias in the elderly. Difficulties in testing the elderly that contribute to this trend of using specific tests rather than an extensive battery include problems with fatigue, visual and auditory impairment, cost, and time. Also, problems regarding lack of norms have been discussed.

The data provided by the WAIS-R are valuable in the diagnosis of Alzheimer's. Other tests that might be considered are the Bender–Gestalt, the Boston Aphasia test, Word Generation tests, Sentence Completion test, Name and Sentence Writing test, and the *Boston Naming Test*. Of course, there are many other instruments that assess such abilities as memory, attention, and concentration, as well as test for aphasia and agnosia. Some of the specific tests which might be used from the Halstead–Reitan Battery include the Category test, which was designed to measure abstract, conceptual, and current learning skill. This test consists of seven subtests and can take the normal subject an hour to complete. The length of this one test alone usually precludes use with the elderly.

The Speech Sounds Perception test requires discrimination between consonant sounds. This test also presents problems for the elderly because of auditory impairment. The Seashore Rhythm test requires the individual to distinguish between two rhythmic patterns. This is a test for nonverbal auditory perception and attention. The Tactual Performance test uses a form board and requires the subject to place forms in ten cut-out spaces with one hand while blindfolded. Again, this test may or may not be applicable when testing an elderly patient—especially one who is suffering from Alzheimer's—in that the test requires an explanation, which probably will not be understood, as well as motor abilities, which may be impaired. The same applies to the Trail Making test, which is a visual-spatial motor test. Again, it is probably more efficient and useful to utilize tests that measure verbal cognitive abilities.

The Reitan–Klove Sensory Perception test is one which can be of value in testing the abilities of the elderly patient. The subtests measure tactile perception, visual field impairments, and auditory acuity.

The Reitan Indiana Aphasia Examination surveys the primary types of aphasia. This test or the Boston Aphasia test should be considered in assessing dementia in the elderly. More is written about the Boston Aphasia test later in this chapter. A neuropsychologist sometimes tests for lateral dominance. This test can also be used to evaluate how well an individual understands directions and can complete tasks. The Halstead Finger Tapping test and Strength of Grip tests are not commonly used in testing for dementia but can be of value in situations of suspected stroke or other forms of brain injury.

As discussed previously, the administration of the complete Halstead–Reitan test is required to obtain a score, allowing for the diagnosis of "normal range" versus "impaired range." In assessing dementia in the elderly, administration of the entire battery is usually not possible or even desirable. The following section is included in order to briefly review some of the other neuropsychological tests that might be considered in testing for dementia and, in particular, Alzheimer's. The qualified neuropsychologist should be familiar with a wide variety of instruments in order to choose the appropriate test for each individual. For example, if there are written expressive language problems suggested when performing the mental status exam, it might be of benefit to administer the Sentence and Name Writing tests or the Sentence Completion test. These tests measure the ability to understand directions and follow commands as well as the ability to express oneself verbally in written language. Organicity is suggested, for example, if an elderly woman who was a school teacher cannot write a coherent sentence. These tests also test for fine motor tremor. The Sentence Completion test requires the individual to complete a sentence from a stem. While the content is important (see Chapter 12), so is the ability to complete the sentence without gross error.

The Benton Visual Retention test is a test of visual construction skill, visual memory, and visual perception. This test is often used rather than the Bender–Gestalt test. The Benton test consists of alternative forms, which allows for retesting without the subjects confounding the results with the practice effect. Test norms are based on age and education; however, these norms may not be of use with the very elderly population. The problem with this test is that there is a tendency to use the results of this one test to diagnose organicity. Again, these tests must be used as part of a more comprehensive diagnostic procedure.

The Visual–Motor Gestalt (Bender–Gestalt) test can be used to test visual perception and comprehension as well as visual memory. The subject is asked to copy nine designs. Immediate visual memory can be tested by having the respondent draw the figures without the cue cards after completing the direct-copy test. Intermediate memory can be tested by having the subject draw the designs after a time delay. The Bender–Gestalt test has been used as a rough screen for organicity, much like the Benton test. The same caution applies. Observing how the subject approaches the task, level of anxiety, and comprehension of directions provides data that are useful in a diagnosis.

The Wechsler Memory test is the most commonly used test of memory. (A number of WAIS-R subtests that are useful in assessing verbal memory are discussed in Chapter 13.) The Wechsler Memory test consists of six subtests. The first test measures orientation and memory. Some of the items such as identifying the year, month, and date are a part of the mental status exam. The second subtest requires the respondent to count, add, and repeat the alphabet within a specific time period.

The third subtest requires the subject to listen to two paragraphs and repeat the details of what they heard. This subtest measures immediate auditory memory and comprehension. The fourth subtest is Digit Span, which is basically the equivalent of the WAIS-R Digit Span test. The Visual Reproduction subtest is a measure of visual memory. The final subtest (Associate Learning) requires the subject to memorize ten word pairs. The Wechsler Memory test is a good device to utilize when assessing the type and extent of memory impairment; however, critics claim that the tests of orientation, information, and mental control are not sensitive to mild brain damage. This is one of the problems in assessing Alzheimer's. Middle- and late-stage Alzheimer's disease is fairly easy to identify, although testing is still important for a differential diagnosis and treatment and management planning. The test also has been criticized because it measures primarily verbal skills. However, this is important in assessing Alzheimer's more so than measuring visual–spatial motor problems.

The *Boston Naming Test* is a test for agnosia that can also be used to evaluate incidental learning and auditory memory. The test consists of sixty pictures of objects and items that the respondent is required to name. The items begin with easily recognized objects, such as a tree and a bed, and increase in difficulty. Stimulus cues are provided if the initial answer is incorrect. Phonetic cues are also provided. A score is arrived at based on the number of correct unassisted and stimulus-cue responses. Incidental learning can be measured by providing the respondent with the name of the items following failure and then returning to the failed items at a later time to see if they are able to retain the information.

Norms are provided; however, these norms are incomplete. For example, the test norms are for adults ages 18 to 59 only. There is a breakdown for ages between 18 and 59 and for schooling; however, the sample size is small. The *Boston Naming Test* is probably best used to gather supportive data rather than as a quantitative instrument.

The Boston Diagnostic Aphasia Examination is a valuable instrument in assessing dementia because of its breadth and depth. The test allows the qualified and trained diagnostician to assess the presence and type of aphasic syndrome, measure the level of performance over a wide range, and make a comprehensive assessment of impairments and spared abilities. This is very important not only in the diagnosis of Alzheimer's but also in the treatment of dementia and in management planning. The areas tested include conversational and expository speech, auditory comprehension, oral expression, understanding written language, and writing. An aphasia severity rating scale is available. The diagnostician can choose appropriate tests and thus limit administrative and assessment time. Some of the subtests are more useful in the assessment of dementia and aphasia than others.

This chapter has focused on neuropsychological assessment concepts and techniques with an emphasis on the need for a comprehensive assessment by a trained and competent professional. Chapter 15 discusses rating scales of functional ability.

CHAPTER 15

Evaluating Functional Ability

An evaluation of functional abilities is an essential part of an assessment. This is related to treatment and management planning. It is important to identify disabilities, limitations, and impairments, as well as spared abilities and skills, in order to help the individual who is suffering to live a full, complete, and satisfying life. This is especially true in cases of dementia. It is essential that the abilities and needs of each individual be identified and that a life situation be developed that will provide the person with as much dignity, autonomy, and independence as possible. Living situation and care decisions must be based on specific and accurate data, regarding not only physical condition but also cognitive abilities and self-care skills. Information about the ability to make rational judgments, abstract reasoning, adaptive skills, and the ability to plan ahead and organize one's day and life is available for a functional and independent living summary if an adequate evaluation has been made.

Chapters 1 and 8 to 15 have discussed the need for a comprehensive and complete evaluation and how each of the procedures and assessment components provide data for an accurate diagnosis regarding dementia. The information obtained from a medical evaluation allows the diagnostician to identify reversible versus irreversible dementias and forms of dementia other than Alzheimer's. The medical examination or history also provides the management care worker or counselor (usually an individual with a background in social services) with information about physical and medical problems and disabilities which might interfere with independent living. With this information, the caseworker can develop a treatment and management plan with arrangement for such services as physical therapy, an auditory or visual exam, or special community services assistance.

The mental status exam is a screening device that identifies areas of impairment and limitations, as well as strengths and spared abilities. As discussed previously, however, more information regarding the extent of these disabilities and abilities is necessary. This information is provided by psychological and neurological testing in many cases. Psychological testing provides the caseworker with data on intellectual abilities as well as emotional status. The next section discusses specific intervention strategies for treating depression, anxiety, acting out, and other emotional and behavioral problems. However, it is important for management personnel to be familiar with personality characteristics and traits and emotional and intellectual problems in the initial management planning phase.

The family interview provides the diagnostician with information regarding chronicity, premorbid abilities, and the nature of cognitive impairments, although, as has been emphasized, quantitative and qualitative information obtained through comprehensive testing is required to determine the exact nature of the impairments and whether they are fixed, likely to progress, or reversible. The family interview is also a valuable source of information about daily living skills and self-care abilities. Talking to the family helps the diagnostician, as well as the case manager, determine the extent and nature of family support systems, interpersonal relations, and unresolved family issues and problems.

The clinical interview allows for the diagnostician to obtain information about thought processes, expressive and receptive language, visual and auditory perceptive ability, emotional state, level of reality testing, and memory functions. Data obtained during the clinical interview can also be of help in management planning. Individuals who are depressed tend to lack goals and have limited motivation and interests. Information about past interests, hobbies, career, and life situation (which is often revealed during the interview) can be used in intervention and treatment.

Various rating scales have been developed not only to aid in the assessment of dementia but also to provide information about specific functional skills. The information on these checklists is usually obtained from a family member. One of the problems with checklists such as these is that they are subjective; however, information obtained in this way can be useful to the case manager. Nursing homes, rehabilitation facilities, and retirement centers usually have checklists of their own that can be used by social workers, physical and occupational therapists, and activity therapists.

Checklists normally include self-maintenance, social functioning, and community living activity:

Self-Maintenance
   Physical functioning
   Personal care and hygiene
   Dressing and grooming
   Nutrition
   Speech and language level
   Eating habits
   Maintenance of personal possessions
   Ability to use medication
   Health maintenance

Social Functioning
   Interaction and involvement with family
   Social skills
   Relationship with friends
   Peer group involvement
   Ability to pursue leisure and recreational activities
   Use of alcohol and other mood-altering substances

Community Living Activities
   Homemaking skills
   Use of transportation
   Ability to shop for self
   Independent travel skill
   Ability to avoid common dangers
   Use of community services

An evaluation of functional abilities commonly would include work-related skills; however, this is not always appropriate because many of the elderly subjects are retired. For general information, the following areas are often evaluated:

Work-Related Skills
   Job-retention behaviors, including tardiness, absenteeism, and work quality
   Relationship skills—peers and supervisors
   Ability to accept responsibility
   Ability to plan and organize
   Personal appearance
   Communication and interviewing skills
   Supervisory skills
   Basic language, writing, and arithmetic skills

CASE #17: RONALD

Ronald is a 76-year-old white male who was in a nursing home when tested. An assessment was recommended because of concerns about his mental abilities and the need to develop plans for the future. Prior to his admission to the nursing facility, he had suffered a diabetic coma and had been unconscious for about eighteen hours. His wife stated that he denied any physical or mental problems and insisted on returning home.

During the interview with the wife, she described her husband as "a brilliant man"; however, she added that he was "very independent." She stated that he had been diagnosed as suffering from diabetes since 1951 and was forced to retire early because of severe disabilities. He had worked as an engineer and held a very responsible and well-paying job with a construction firm.

The wife reported that her husband has suffered from a number of diabetic seizures and produced photos of him lying on the floor following episodes. It was becoming evident that the wife was very submissive and that her husband's denial was a real issue with her. In planning for the future, this issue must be discussed, with Ronald accepting the fact that he does indeed suffer from a debilitating disorder and needs some form of professional help and care.

The wife continued that as her husband's physical problems became more severe, he became more dependent and demanding. He also does not adhere to medical advice about diet and health. The wife stated that medical sources diagnosed the husband as "a brittle diabetic." She stated that during one seizure episode, he broke his hip. During another, he burned his forehead when he fell on a lightbulb.

The wife reported that her husband was beginning to have problems with memory and concentration. She added that, in her opinion, he was also "very depressed." During the clinical interview, the subject denied most of the reports given by his wife. He stated that he had "no problems" prior to the last six months. However, testing indicated that indeed he was aware of his physical problems and that he was angry, frightened, and depressed. Testing also indicated that he was a very controlling and egocentric individual who became easily frustrated and irritated. These characterological factors make any illness intolerable.

The neuropsychological assessment suggested that the subject does have problems with focus, memory, and attention. Expressive and receptive language abilities were intact, although he does tend to be preoccupied, tangential, and circumstantial. There also appeared to be problems with judgment, incremental learning, and analytical ability. Orientation was poor. At times, he confabulated. Recall for words was poor, with signs of mild agnosia. When asked to write a sentence, he wrote, "I am presently presenting my diabetic reaction in regard to my improvement here at the nursing home." The subject had problems with the *Boston Naming Test* as well as a number of the Boston Aphasia subtests. He does not listen well and had problems attending. There was some indication of a hearing loss. Tactile abilities were intact, although he had problems with fine motor skills. This was due, in part, to a poorly healed broken wrist. Ambulation was impaired. He is a frail man who walks with a cane. Balance and equilibrium were poor.

He was able to read and understand sentences and commands. Responses to the BDI indicated that he was moderately to severely depressed.

The diagnosis was dementia due to multiple etiologies (rather than Alzheimer's) and major depression—single episode (moderate to severe).

Using the functional checklist from the previous section, the following evaluation can be made:

Self-Maintenance

Physical functioning: Limited ambulatory ability with risk of falling; risk of future diabetic seizures with possibility of severe physical injury

Personal care and hygiene: Needs help with bathing and toileting; difficulty in dressing and grooming

Nutrition: Unable to plan and prepare own meals; tendency to disregard medical advice regarding diet; poor nutrition adds to risk of diabetic reactions

Speech and language: Abilities intact but shows poor judgment and does not listen to others well; in denial about medical and emotional problems

Maintenance of possessions and autonomy: Depends on wife for basic needs; limited ability to plan for the future

Ability to use medication and provide for health care: Denial results in noncompliance

Social Functioning

Interaction with family: Tends to be demanding, dependent, and domineering

Social skills: Limited social involvement; preoccupied with health problems

Relationship with friends: Few friends; depends on wife and family

Peer group involvement: Very limited

Ability to pursue leisure and recreational activities: Physical disabilities and depression have resulted in his being very isolated and withdrawn

Use of alcohol: Denied by subject and wife

Community Activities

Home living skills: Limited; relies on wife

Use of transportation: Limited; tends to become confused and disoriented; physical disabilities limit ambulation

Ability to shop for self: Limited

Use of community services: Resists involvement or use

Work-Related Skills

Not applicable

Recommendations included helping the subject realize and accept the fact that he has a serious and debilitating disease and that he must comply with medical advice. A consultation with his physician was arranged. It was also stressed that at the time of the assessment, he needed intensive care. He and his wife were advised to discuss this with the aid of a therapist. The woman needed support and help in dealing with her own feelings of concern for the future and her codependency.

It was suggested that antidepressant medication and therapy might improve his mood. The cognitive problems did not appear to be progressive and might clear up with time. As the individual's functional, emotional, and physical problems diminish, plans might be made for returning home with the help of in-home community services. While in the nursing home, the individual was encouraged to become more active and socially involved. The staff, physical therapy personnel, and social services department became involved in the treatment and management planning.

Part III discusses treatment, management, family, and legal issues.

TREATMENT AND MANAGEMENT OF THE DEMENTIAS

CHAPTER 16

Treatment of the Dementias

Gene May Speed Alzheimer's Fight
Memory Tests May Help Gauge Alzheimer's Risk
New Clues Found on Causes of Alzheimer's
Experiments Suggest Link between Zinc, Alzheimer's
Drugs Help Buy Time against Alzheimer's
New Drug Gives Hope to Alzheimer's Patients

These were headlines in major newspapers during one week. Alzheimer's disease is a devastating, nonreversible, progressive, organic disease that affects between 2.5 and 4 million Americans. The media as well as the general public clamor for news of a cure or at least a way to slow down the symptoms of Alzheimer's. As of January 1996, there is no cure for Alzheimer's. Publicity and media focus on the disorder has been of benefit in that it alerts the public to signs and symptoms which hopefully will result in early detection. However, as this book points out, it is primary that a diagnosis be complete and comprehensive. There is no "quick test" for Alzheimer's disease.

A comprehensive evaluation will identify reversible forms of dementia and allow treatment. Chapters 17 and 18 discuss use of psychotropic medications and psychotherapy to treat psychosis, depression, and anxiety. These emotional disorders often present symptoms of dementia. Treatment of medical disorders with symptoms of dementia alleviates these symptoms.

However, no drug or procedure has been developed to "cure" Alzheimer's or even arrest the progress of the disease. Brain atrophy cannot be reversed. The only drug which has been approved for Alzheimer's is tacrine. At present, 50,000 people are taking this medication, which, according to reports, has limited ability to slow progress of the disease. This medication has been used in early-stage Alzheimer's. The drug increases the level of the neurotransmitter acetylcholine (ACh).

The major focus of research at this time is on neurotransmitter deficits. (As discussed earlier, structural damage cannot be reversed.) The hypothesis that a cholinergic deficit impairs learning and memory has been documented over the last twenty years. Interventions are based on enhancing cholinergic neurotransmission.

One of the strategies suggested is to administer ACh therapy precursors, primarily choline and lecithin. However, the results of ACh therapy has not been significantly beneficial. Cholinergic antagonists, including RS-86 bethanechol, arecoline, oxotremorine, and nicotine, have been used in experiments.

A third approach has been to use cholinesterase inhibitors since enhancement strategies have not proved to be beneficial. These include physostigmine and tetrahydroaminoacridine.

Because of evidence of decreased levels of noradrenaline and dopamine in Alzheimer's patients, monoaminergic drugs have also been tested. However, as is the case in most of these interventions, enhancement of neurotransmitters does not change the basic cause of the deficiency, which is related to neuronal loss.

Pharmacological approaches which are not neurotransmitter specific have also been used. In these cases, it is suggested that the secondary causes of cognitive impairment are actually being treated, which is of value but not a cure for Alzheimer's. Similarly, medical treatment of illnesses which present as Alzheimer's does not "cure" Alzheimer's. In the event of a coexisting disorder such as cardiovascular disease, respiratory problems, and other systemic disorders, treatment is important.

Many geriatric patients present symptoms of fatigue, psychomotor retardation, and lack of motivation. Amphetamines have been used in these cases. (See Chapter 17 regarding side effects and cautions in using amphetamine therapy with the elderly.) Specific medications used have included pentylenetetrazol, pipradrol, and pemoline. A review of the literature suggests no benefit to Alzheimer's patients.

Early researchers suggested that Alzheimer's might be related to decreased blood flow to the brain. While this may be a coexisting disorder with Alzheimer's, reduced blood flow is not a causal factor of Alzheimer's. However, cerebral vasodilators are used to treat the coexisting disorder.

Nootropic drugs, or "cognitive enhancers," including piracetam, have been used in an attempt to improve memory, alertness, and socialization. However, the benefit of this medication has not been documented.

One of the major problems in evaluating the effectiveness of the drugs currently being promised in the press as "cures" for Alzheimer's is that the drug studies appear to have major flaws. In many cases, the sample sizes are small and research conditions uncontrolled. Also, many researchers do not differentiate between different types of dementia. It could well be that cases of improved cognition are among those patients who are not suffering from Alzheimer's disease.

Research continues in such areas as nerve growth, neuronal tissue transplants, and genetic intervention. Funding for this research has increased from $50 million in 1986 to $295 million in 1993. The most promising area of research is to develop a way to treat the disease before the degenerative process has advanced. Structural damage cannot be repaired or reversed. This emphasizes the need for accurate and early diagnosis. Neurochemical, neuroendocrinological, and brain imaging have not proved to be reliable diagnostic tools to date. However, brain-behavior diagnosis, where cognitive impairments and deficits are identified, allows for one to differentiate between the reversible and the irreversible dementias and provides information regarding treatment and management of the functional and behavioral problems.

CHAPTER 17

The Use of Psychotropic Drugs in Treatment

At present, no effective treatment has been developed or discovered to reverse the cognitive impairments associated with Alzheimer's disease. However, psychotropic drugs (those drugs which effect mood and behavior) have been developed and are currently being used to effectively treat emotional and psychological illnesses such as depression, anxiety, and schizophrenia. Chapter 18 discusses how psychotherapy and psychotropic drugs are often used concurrently in the treatment of mental illness.

Medical treatment and intervention are also used to treat many physical diseases and illnesses that present symptoms similar to Alzheimer's. This book has emphasized the need for a complete and accurate diagnosis to differentiate between the reversible dementias and Alzheimer's.

This chapter focuses primarily on the use of psychotropic drugs to treat illnesses of the elderly and special considerations with those suffering from dementia. One of the problems encountered in using psychotropic drugs with the elderly, especially in cases of dementia, is the lack of controlled studies. While general principles apply, there appears to be a lack of scientific data regarding the efficiency and effect of many of the medications on elderly patients. This is due, in part, to wide differences in physical health and factors brought about by age-related phenomena. There are significant differences in the same-age population because of differences in state of health. In testing hundreds of individuals from the age of 65 to 101, this examiner has discovered not only extensive differences in the level of cognition and functioning but also extensive differences in general health. Diseases, injuries, systemic failures, and nutritional factors all affect the way medications are absorbed, distributed, and metabolized. The need for monitoring the effect and side effect of psychotropic medications (as well as other medications) is primary because of the danger of side effects, especially toxicity. The synergetic effects of the drugs must also be considered.

In the elderly, lean muscle and body water tend to decrease, while body fat increases. Psychotropic drugs, which are lipophilic, will be more widely distributed than lithium carbonate (used to treat bipolar disorder). Reduced efficiency of the liver can result in drugs remaining in the system for a longer period of time, possibility resulting in toxicity. Low-potency neuroleptic drugs tend to be eliminated more slowly than high-potency neuroleptics. Disturbance of renal functions can be further reduced by diuretics. Drugs with anticholinergic properties can increase confusion and memory problems in the elderly, especially those suffering from dementia. These issues are discussed in more detail later. However, from a global standpoint, it can be stated that monitoring of the side effects of all kinds of medications with the elderly and treatment by physicians aware of special considerations and issues regarding the elderly are essential.

Family members should ask the following questions regarding medication of an elderly significant other. If the answers to these questions are not specific and direct, a second opinion should be considered, just as a second opinion should be considered if a loved one is diagnosed as suffering from Alzheimer's after a brief interview and examination:

1. Why is this medication prescribed?
2. What are the desired effects? How are these effects to be monitored and by whom?
3. Are there other forms of treatment?
4. What are the risks and side effects?
5. What are the interactions with other medications currently being used?
6. How will changes in health and physical conditions change the effectiveness and the side effects?
7. For how long will this medication be used, and how often will its use be reviewed?
8. What will be the cost of these drugs, and are there generic forms available?

Recently, there has been an emphasis on reducing the use of drugs, in general, and, more specifically, psychotropic medications in nursing homes and similar facilities. A distinction must be made between the use of psychotropic medications to treat mental illnesses that are primary, such as depression, and the use of psychotropic medications to control behavioral symptoms, such as agitation and acting out.

The elderly, like others in the general population, can suffer from depression, anxiety, or psychosis. These illnesses or conditions can be primary or coexist with dementia. Again, effective treatment requires an accurate diagnosis regarding chronicity, cause, degree, and course. A number of cases have been presented discussing primary emotional disorders misdiagnosed as dementia. Antidepressant medication and psychotherapy have been suggested as appropriate treatments for depression. However, the particular antidepressant and dosage must be considered based on the physical and mental condition and state of the patient.

Psychotropic medications have also been used to control the behavior of those individuals who are suffering from Alzheimer's and to treat specific symptoms such as sleep disturbance, wandering, agitation, and aggressiveness. Chapter 18 discusses the use of psychological and behavioral techniques to control or treat these behaviors.

This chapter focuses primarily on general principles in the use of psychotropic medications, side effects, and cautions. The following cases are presented to illustrate the difference between responsible use of psychotropic medication and lack of adequate consideration regarding the synergetic effect of other drugs, the need for medication, adequate monitoring of side effects, and responsible review of treatment. Too often, symptoms are observed and medications prescribed without adequate knowledge of the causal factors.

Recently, a national newspaper ran a headline "Test for Suicide Risks." The article stated that a study from Johns Hopkins University found that medical doctors could detect the risk of suicide in their patients by asking four simple questions. According to the article, these questions related to feelings of "guilt and hopelessness, depressed mood and sleep disturbance." Risk of suicide and major depression cannot be evaluated by asking four questions; yet many elderly patients are asked if they "feel depressed" and, if the answer is affirmative, prescribed antidepressant medication. The same is often true with anxiety and the resulting prescription of an antianxiety medication. Antianxiety medication tends to be addictive, has severe withdrawal symptoms, and can create paradoxical excitement. Too often, a review of these prescriptions is not made and side effects such as ataxia (falling down) judged to be related to "old age."

CASE #18: HAROLD

Harold was 87 years old when assessed. He had been living in a nursing home for about six months. Prior to that, he had lived with his daughter. Admission to the nursing home was precipitated by emotional and physical problems. The individual had suffered a stroke and was partially paralyzed. An interview with the daughter and a functional-abilities evaluation indicated that he was unable to bathe or dress himself, was incontinent, had problems with executive functions such as planning and organizing his life and his activities, and was unable to eat without assistance. The daughter and staff at the nursing home verified the fact that he had more recently become agitated, more confused, and aggressive. He slept during much of the day and then shouted and wandered at night.

He was on a variety of medications for pain, arthritis, and congestive heart failure. A review of his medical chart indicated that on admission to the nursing home, he had been prescribed a low dosage of a low-potency neuroleptic medication. Two weeks later, he had been prescribed another neuroleptic. About six weeks later, he was prescribed a third neuroleptic. The first two neuroleptics were not discontinued. The dosages of the three neuroleptics were well below therapeutic dosage levels, even for an elderly patient. The subject had also been prescribed an antidepressant, sedative medication, and antianxiety medication. As time went by, he began falling down and became more agitated, assaultive, and aggressive. His cognitive and functional disabilities increased, and he began to hallucinate. He was judged to be suffering from "late-stage Alzheimer's" and spent most of his time restrained in a gerichair. His family was amazed at his rapid deterioration physically, functionally, and mentally. Independently, they requested an assessment for Alzheimer's.

CASE #19: ALICE

Alice was 77 years old when assessed. She was admitted to a rehabilitation facility following a hip injury. Prior to that time, she had lived in an independent living residential facility. On arrival at the rehabilitation center, she was placed in a unit for individuals who needed intensive physical care. However, as she improved, she was moved to a unit that allowed her more independence and autonomy. Initially, she had displayed symptoms of depression. She identified a number of issues that were bothering her, including fear of not being able to live independently, loss of a brother earlier in the year, reliance on family for care, and financial problems. The individual did not have a history of depression and was not judged to be suicidal. During an assessment, her ability to plan and organize was observed to be intact. Expressive and receptive language skills were well developed. Prior to her hip injury, she had been very active and socially involved. She expressed an interest in creative arts and became involved readily in the social activities at the facility. She was motivated to attend physical and occupational therapy.

Initially, it was considered to prescribe an antidepressant. However, she responded well to psychotherapy (where she talked about her concerns and feelings) and involvement in social activities and events.

She became more outgoing and less anxious. Previously, she had problems sleeping. However, her sleep-disturbance problems abated as her mood improved. The staff at the facility, her physician, and family all cooperated in her treatment program. In retrospect, it was agreed that her depression and anxiety were situational and that the decision not to use antidepressant and antianxiety medication had been a wise decision.

According to studies, certain classes of drugs should be avoided or used in minimal doses when treating elderly patients with dementia. Alzheimer's disease is related to a cholinergic deficit. Alzheimer's patients are susceptible to increased confusion, disorientation, and memory problems when treated with drugs with anticholinergic side effects. Some psychotropic medications also have sedative, hypotension, extrapyramidal, and cardiotoxicity side effects. At random, prescription of medication without experience in geriatric pharmacology and lack of monitoring of side effects can result in seriously detrimental side effects, such as in the case with Harold (see Case #18). The important factor to realize in prescribing psychotropic medication for the elderly patient (especially where there are signs of dementia) is that the basic pharmacological principles apply but that special considerations must be taken in the determination of the dosage as well as the specific medications used.

It is beyond the scope of this book to discuss specific side effects, dosages for the elderly, synergetic effects, and monitoring techniques. In brief, general side effects for antipsychotic (neuroleptic), antianxiety (minor tranquilizers), and antidepressant medications will be mentioned.

Antidepressants with high sedation, hypotension, anticholinergic, and cardiotoxicity side effects include amitriptyline, imipramine, and doxepin. Neuroleptics with high sedation, hypotension, and anticholinergic side effects include chlorpromazine and thioridazine. Trifluoperazine, thiothixene, and haloperidol are low on these side effects but tend to have extrapyramidal side effects. Extrapyramidal side effects can be countered with an anti-Parkinson drug. For agitation, anxiety, and restlessness, a low dosage of a high-potency neuroleptic (such as the last three mentioned) tends to be the drug of choice on a prn basis. Antianxiety medications are generally not used with the elderly—especially in cases of dementia—because of their tendency to cloud sensorium, impair memory, and produce ataxia. A stable environment with limited stimulation and psychotherapy to address the anxious patient's fears and concerns tends to be more effective and of less risk than using antianxiety medication. The same basic principle of not using medication to treat sleep disturbances applies. Chapters 18 and 21 discuss psychotherapy and dealing with specific behavioral and management problems.

CHAPTER 18

Psychological Treatment

All my family and friends are dead. I have no one to tell about my pain.
                    —Statement by an 80-year-old woman
                    during a clinical interview

The emotional and psychological problems of the elderly are probably undertreated. This is especially true in the case of Alzheimer's patients. During early- and middle-stage Alzheimer's (see Chapter 19), individuals suffering from the disease still have some cognitive capacities; and attempts can and should be made to address their emotional problems and concerns. Early- and middle-stage Alzheimer's patients tend to experience feelings of confusion, anger, denial, and fear. They are aware of problems with memory and orientation during these stages. Their fears, however, are often undisclosed and unaddressed. This results in more anxiety and internal tension, adding to increased functional disability. When one is anxious and afraid, his or her ability to think and function tends to decrease. In the case of chronic anxiety, this is especially disabling.

One of the reasons that Alzheimer's patients do not receive adequate psychological treatment and care is that the patient tends to present as uncooperative and resistant. This is because, during early-stage Alzheimer's, there are commonly attempts to confabulate and hide the disability. Also, elderly people are often unsure of the psychological process and consider talking to "strangers" intrusive. They usually feel vulnerable and dislike scrutiny just like the rest of us, even though identifying their fears, concerns, and problems can lead to alleviation of depression and anxiety.

Another reason that the elderly and Alzheimer's patients tend to be undertreated is the general belief that there is no help or benefit. Just as individuals with Alzheimer's tend not to receive the benefit of regular visual and auditory examinations, caretakers often have the attitude that therapy will be of little value. It is common to focus on the basic health and hygiene needs of the Alzheimer's patient, with little attention given to feelings. Agitation and acting out behaviors are controlled, in many cases, by psychotropic drugs rather than addressing the causal factors. (See Chapters 20 and 21 on management of Alzheimer's patients by structuring the environment and through behavior-modification methods.)

This common belief that psychological services will not benefit the Alzheimer's patient extends to thinking about the benefits of a complete evaluation. As discussed previously, this is inexcusable. A significant number of the individuals assessed by this examiner who had been diagnosed as suffering from Alzheimer's were not. False positives lead to incalculable pain for the individual patient and gross mismanagement.

A third reason that Alzheimer's patients are not provided with psychological services is because of the tendency (and this may be a global and possibly inaccurate statement) for mental health professionals to want to treat a rather healthy population with the hope for recovery. Many individuals, especially the young in our youth-oriented society, have reservations about dealing with "old people." There is little question that the treatment settings, including the geriatric units of hospitals and Alzheimer's sections of nursing homes, are depressing and often chaotic. However, there is also a sense of joy related to holding the hand of an 83-year-old woman who is unable to talk or communicate well but responds to the attention, respect, and love provided her during an evaluation or in therapy.

A fourth reason that the elderly, especially Alzheimer's patients, do not receive psychological services is that the helping profession is just now beginning to realize the need for these services and set up training programs. The major reason that I am writing this book is to share my experiences over the last seven or eight years of working with the elderly, especially in the field of assessment and the evaluation of dementia in the elderly.

A fifth reason that the elderly do not obtain adequate psychological help is related to money, although this is changing. Medicare and Medicaid do provide funds for the assessment and treatment of the elderly in most cases. In fact, some states require that nursing homes reevaluate individuals with psychological problems annually. Until the need for a complete initial evaluation is realized, many individuals who have severe emotional problems are not identified. Again, violent acting out tends to attract attention; however, the severely depressed or anxious elderly resident—especially if he or she is also suffering from some form of dementia—is not normally treated or assisted.

It has been estimated that 16 to 20 million Americans suffer from major depression each year. An even greater number suffer from anxiety disorders. Over 2 million individuals have been diagnosed as schizophrenic. Thirteen percent of the population abuses alcohol or other mood-altering drugs. From 2.5 to 4 million individuals suffer form some form of dementia. As discussed earlier, emotional illnesses too often are diagnosed as Alzheimer's; however, there are many cases based on the aforementioned statistics where an emotional illness preexists or is coexistent with Alzheimer's. The fact that many elderly individuals have emotional illnesses that can be treated is one reason that the elderly should be allowed psychological services—first, to diagnose or identify reversible forms of dementia and treat these disorders, and second, to diagnose and treat emotional disorders that coexist with Alzheimer's. An individual who suffers from Alzheimer's and depression or Alzheimer's and generalized anxiety disorder is likely to be more dysfunctional than one who suffers from only an emotional disorder or Alzheimer's. An emotional disorder tends to exacerbate cognitive and functional problems.

The same is true in the case of a coexisting personality disorder. Management is more difficult when the individual is basically antisocial. Old age does not improve compatibility and social skills. In fact, we tend to become more vulnerable and our adaptive skills less adequate as we age.

The elderly tend to have common emotional and psychological problems related to life-stage situations and events. There appears to be a common element of loss which is related to loss of health, physical problems, loss of roles and purpose in life, and loss of loved ones and support systems. This varies based on particulars and the individual, as discussed in Chapter 4. Some individuals age more successfully than others, although they have suffered losses, pain, and negative circumstances.

Nevertheless, depression is common in the elderly. This is one reason that an assessment of mood and emotional state is important in making an evaluation. The symptoms of major depression are, in many cases, similar to those of dementia, including problems with memory, attention and concentration, and orientation.

Responses to the BDI and the BHS tend to reflect feelings of anhedonia, negative thoughts about the future, and unremitting feelings of sadness. A common response of the more severely depressed is, "I have thoughts of killing myself but would not carry them out."

CASE #20: DORIS

Doris was 77 years old when assessed. She entered a nursing home following treatment for addiction to a prescription antianxiety medication. It is not uncommon for the elderly to mismanage their prescription medications, sometimes with severe side effects. It is interesting and an example of medical mismanagement that, at the time of this assessment, she had been prescribed another major tranquilizer for her anxiety.

Doris had been a resident for about six months but was not adapting to community living. She refused to enter into social activities and spent most of her time isolated in her room. Her level of energy was low. The staff reported that she appeared to have problems with concentration and was beginning to "talk to herself." Alzheimer's disease was suspected. She had problems with hearing; however, no effort had been made to arrange for an evaluation of auditory abilities.

During the clinical interview, data about her life were revealed. It had been reported that her 56-year-old son had died of cancer while she was in the hospital being treated for her addiction. The closeness and dependent nature of her relationship with the son soon became apparent. The woman had lived with the son for the last twenty years following the death of her husband. The son had never married. Mother and son spent most of their time together. Their lives were closely intertwined. Social activities and interactions outside of the relationship were limited. The son did not date. Mother did the cooking and housekeeping. The son was responsible for the financial well-being of the couple. The mother stated that following her discharge from the hospital and admission to the nursing home, distant relatives sold the house and all of her belongings. She added that she had not even been allowed to bring her treasured items into the nursing home because her granddaughter "kept everything."

During the assessment, the individual showed problems with memory. Concentration was poor because of her emotional state. She was suffering from severe depression. She had not been allowed to grieve the loss of her son, the loss of her role as a valuable person to someone else, the loss of her addictive drug (which is one of the often unrecognized issues in treating chemical dependency), and the loss of her home and her belongings. She was not suffering from Alzheimer's.

A recommendation was made for psychotherapy. She was encouraged to join a group on grief and grieving. The granddaughter was persuaded to give her back a chest of drawers and her collection of porcelain figurines, which she now displays on a shelf in her room. Doris, it was discovered, had the ability to play the piano. Her therapist encouraged her to play—at first, alone, and later, for other residents. Most nursing and retirement settings have pianos available for the benefit of residents.

In therapy, the loss issues and concerns about the future were discussed. The subject is passive dependent with avoidant personality traits but was encouraged to become more self-sufficient and sociable. She found a fellow resident who has similar interests and spends some time with her, although she is still moderately isolative and withdrawn. The staff reports that she is less "forgetful" and "at times, even smiles." The antianxiety medication has been discontinued. She is currently on a low dosage of antidepressant medication which is nonaddictive. It is probable that, without therapy, her condition would have continued to deteriorate.

Family therapy is often of benefit for individuals who are suffering from depression due to loss, especially in the case of a spouse or other loved one. This allows the whole family to go through the grief process.

CASE #21: SALLY

Sally was living in a retirement center when assessed. She was 90 years old. Except for problems with vision, she was physically able. Her vision had been corrected to some extent by glasses; however, she still had to use a magnifying glass to read.

About two years ago, prior to the assessment, she and her husband had lived out of state. Their son had encouraged the couple to move closer to him and his family. The apartment in the retirement home was attractively furnished with the couple's belongings from their previous life. About six months after their move, the husband died. Sally was not allowed to resolve her grief and go through the steps of grieving. Her family told her to be "brave" and reminded her that she and her husband had experienced sixty-four years of marriage.

During the assessment, the woman was encouraged to talk about her life with her husband. It was painful for her. It appeared that this was the first time that she had been allowed to cry. The "assessment" continued for more than three hours, with the resident bringing out pictures, mementos, and letters. She also talked about how difficult it was to relocate and give up her church and friends. The assessment provided data not only on her cognitive and functional abilities but also on her emotional status. It also provided her with an opportunity to begin the healing process. Arrangements were made for individual as well as family therapy.

It was suggested that the son and his family join the woman and share their personal experiences and feelings about their relationship with their father and grandfather. Disclosing and sharing feelings and emotions rather than repressing them leads to resolution.

The woman was also encouraged to begin a "life review" with the help of a therapist. This technique allows an individual to review their own successes and failures as well as goals, relationships, joys, and sorrows. The individual is instructed to use a tape recorder. This can then be written up as a family history and shared with family members. Therapeutically, a life review tends to provide feelings of accomplishment and hope rather than negativity. It also prepares one for a healthy transition.

CASE #22: JUNE

June is suffering from middle- to late-stage dementia of the Alzheimer's type as well as schizophrenia. Prior to the assessment, she was not taking any antipsychotic medication. The staff reported "odd and unusual" behavior; however, the assessment, a review of the medical records, and an interview with the family clearly indicated that her psychosis was chronic and schizophrenic. Schizophrenia increased the patient's cognitive and functional problems. While she was able to answer a few simple questions, there was evidence of disorganized thought processes and behavior. At times, she became incoherent. On other occasions, she lost track of what she was doing and saying. She thought that the examiner was her son. She was not particularly depressed. Throughout the assessment, she kept smiling and laughed inappropriately. During one period of coherency, she stated that "little boys" come to visit her. She continued, "They talk to me. They don't hurt me. They are very nice to me." She then laughed again and said, "I like this place, Bill."

Neuroleptic medication was prescribed. The staff reported some improvement in comprehension and the ability to communicate; however, middle- to late-stage Alzheimer's disabilities continued, including problems with memory, orientation, and cognition.

Adequate treatment and care requires recognizing not only strengths and weaknesses, abilities, and disabilities but also needs. In these cases, an accurate assessment was required to provide the psychological and pharmacological services that would benefit the individual. Treatment possibilities included individual, group, and family therapy as well as psychotropic medication. Major improvements were seen in the cognitive and functional abilities of the first two individuals, with slight improvement in the third case.

CHAPTER 19

Communicating with Alzheimer's Patients

It is important to recognize that communication problems arise when interrelating with individuals suffering from Alzheimer's disease. These problems are related to specific deficits and disabilities common in Alzheimer's. The severity and nature of the specific deficit varies from individual to individual as well as during the course of the disease.

Failure to recognize the nature of the disability results in problems in diagnosis, treatment, management, and care. It is of benefit for all of those who interact with individuals with Alzheimer's to be aware of overcoming these communication barriers and problems. Failure to communicate as clearly and accurately as possible with the person suffering from Alzheimer's will result in poor treatment and care, as well as frustration on the part of the caretaker and the patient.

The ability to understand and be understood varies during the progressive stages of Alzheimer's. During the early stage, the sufferer tends to recognize the communication failure and inability to understand and be understood. This leads to frustration, irritation, anxiety, and often anger. Family members and other caretakers also become irritated, frustrated, and angry. Having to repeat the same command many times or answer the same question is one of the most common complaints of caretakers. Failure to complete a task or remember that a question has been answered is related to problems with memory and is not volitional in the case of the individual with Alzheimer's. This must be recognized. Suggestions follow on how to compensate for specific disabilities and problems in communication.

First, it is appropriate to discuss the basic principles of communication and possible problem areas. Communication can be considered as a loop with a message sent through time and space to a receiver. To complete the loop, the receiver becomes the transmitter, again sending or returning a message over time and space to the original sender. Language and communication theorists suggest that disturbance can occur in various places during the process.

There may be problems in the initial transmission. These problems can vary in nature. The individual who is speaking might not be speaking loudly enough or be speaking in a language not completely understood by the intended receiver. Individuals with Alzheimer's often regress. In one particular assessment, an 80-year-old Hispanic patient appeared to understand English. However, as the procedure continued, it became obvious that she was beginning to think in her native language. Thus, the sender of a message must be sure that the message is clear, concise, and transmitted in a way that, in all likelihood, can be received.

Disturbance or "noise," as communication experts say, can develop in the transmittal line. Lack of attention or concentration by the intended receiver can result in poor communication. This is why it is important to make sure that environmental factors do not interfere with communication. A noisy or chaotic environment not only interferes with communication with the individual suffering from Alzheimer's but also can create additional anxiety and, in some cases, a catastrophic response. A catastrophic response is one in which the individual becomes overwhelmed or decompensates. This often happens in situations where demand is greater than capacity. Asking the Alzheimer's patient to carry out three-stage tasks can become overwhelming. Providing more information than can be assimilated can result in overload.

A third problem area in the communication loop can develop with the intended receiver. We have already discussed how auditory problems can result in failure to receive a message. Problems with receptive language as well as abstract reasoning are common in Alzheimer's disease. While the message may be clear, simple, and precise and disturbance minimized, it is still very possible for the patient not to understand the message.

Expressive language problems, the ability to retrieve information, problems with word finding, and problems with attention and abstract reasoning can all interfere with the return message when the receiver becomes the sender. How common it is for a family member to comment that they thought the Alzheimer's sufferer understood a message only to receive a nonsense or completely incoherent or incongruent reply.

As in the original transmission of the message, noise can interfere with communication in the last stage of the loop. The caretaker, diagnostician, clinician, or family member may not be attentive or may misunderstand the meaning of the message. Often, individuals with

Alzheimer's disease are misunderstood because the real message is not perceived by the receiver. It is necessary to attempt to understand the needs and situation of the Alzheimer's patient. Often, they are frightened, confused, anxious, or angry (or any combination of these). When an Alzheimer's sufferer continually asks for a dead spouse or parent, they are expressing a fear. Confrontation or attempting to improve this sense of reality is usually useless and counterproductive. Assuring the person that their security and dependency needs will be met is a better approach.

Last, there may be problems with the original sender, such as a hearing loss or language or comprehension problems of their own. Often, family members are overwhelmed and frustrated. It is not uncommon for there to be unresolved emotional issues, which can lead to misunderstanding, with failure to adequately and accurately comprehend the returned message.

Alzheimer's sufferers tend to have common symptoms that interfere with communication. Although the severity of these symptoms or problems may vary, problems related to age and emotional state are likely. Individuals who suffer from Alzheimer's disease are not necessarily spared the degenerative disabilities of old age. Vision and hearing problems, as well motoric disabilities, are common. In one particular assessment, an individual could not speak because of a stroke. He also could not write. Methods had to be devised to adequately and accurately assess cognitive abilities, such as the capacity to abstract, reason, and problem solve. This particular individual had been assessed as suffering from vascular dementia. However, a more complete examination determined that many executive functions and mental abilities had been spared. This illustrates the need for a comprehensive assessment detailing impaired as well as spared abilities.

Alzheimer's patients tend to be depressed and anxious during the early stages, although as the disorder continues, there is a tendency to become less depressed. During middle-stage Alzheimer's, acting out behavior is common. These emotions and emotional states can exacerbate communication problems and must be considered along with physical disabilities when trying to communicate with loved ones suffering from Alzheimer's.

Specific problems experienced by those suffering from Alzheimer's include problems with orientation, memory, attention and concentration, expressive language, receptive language, abstract thinking, incremental learning, and organization and planning. To improve communication, it is of benefit to judge the extent of each of these disabilities and attempt to compensate for them.

Problems with orientation result in confusion and agitation. Memory problems interfere with task completion and assimilation of new information. Because those with Alzheimer's are commonly disoriented and have problems adapting to new situations, change results in anxiety and agitation. Moving a treasured object or changing the furniture in a room can result in an unexpected catastrophic response.

As previously discussed, problems with language (aphasia and agnosia) increase communication problems, as do problems with attention and concentration. Communication is complicated by problems with abstract reasoning, judgment, problem solving, and reality testing.

Understanding the various stages of Alzheimer's and the related impairments and disabilities is important in communication and management. One reason that a complete assessment—including areas of reasoning, language, memory, and orientation—is necessary is to determine which abilities have been spared and how to use these abilities in communication and relating in an appropriate caring and loving way. Tracking changes in abilities and disabilities should be made over time and techniques and strategies of communication and management adapted.

Alzheimer's disease is a progressive degenerative disease. Because the disorder is progressive and because symptoms vary in type and severity between individuals, it is difficult to identify specific stages and demarcation between stages. Thus, the following stages are guidelines:

Stage 1—No Cognitive Decline

Stage 2—Initial Cognitive Decline

    Individual recognizes some memory problems with expressed concern

    Loses or misplaces items

    Forgets names

    No problems in social or career functioning

Stage 3—Mild Cognitive Decline

    Problems recalling details

    Some confusion and disorientation in demanding social and work problems

    Reports from co-workers of performance problems

    Problems in finding names and words

    Loss of direction when traveling in unfamiliar areas

    Increased anxiety and denial to compensate for fears

Stage 4—Moderate Cognitive Decline

    Specific defects more evident

    Problems with attention and concentration

    Problems with immediate and intermediate memory; long-term memory may be intact

    Problems in handling personal finances

Continues to be oriented with time; recognizes familiar faces and places
Can travel to familiar locations but withdraws from challenging situations
May become defensive in denial

Stage 5—Moderately Severe Cognitive Decline
Individual forgets addresses, names, and phone numbers
Self-care abilities decline because of problems in carrying out tasks
Problems with orientation
Hygiene and dressing problems but usually able to eat and toilet by self

Stage 6—Severe Cognitive Decline
Forgets spouse's name
Long-term memory and fund of knowledge impairment
Disoriented in regard to place, time, and situation
Sleep disturbance
Personality change with possible delusions and repetitive behaviors
Anxiety, agitation, and acting out are common
Apathy tends to follow with isolation and lack of energy

Stage 7—Very Severe Cognitive Decline
Inability to communicate
Incontinence
Complete care required; cannot feed self; often unable to walk
Vegetative state and more specific and focal neurological symptoms

Specific suggestions related to communicating with Alzheimer's patients include the following:

1. Identify the specific deficits and attempt to compensate for them.
2. Improve sensory impairments. Often, Alzheimer's patients are not evaluated for visual or auditory disabilities. While an evaluation may be difficult and require a diagnostician with special skill, remediation of these problems will improve functioning and communication, especially in the early stages of Alzheimer's.
3. Be nonconfrontive when dealing with delusions and problems in reality testing. Arguing does not improve cognition. In the case of insistence that a dead spouse or parent exists, it often helps to allow the person with Alzheimer's to discuss past happy events and the relationship. Reviewing pictures of the person is often therapeutic.
4. Continue to treat the person with dignity and feelings of autonomy and personal control. Persuasion is better than giving orders, especially during early-stage Alzheimer's.
5. Be direct in communication. Make sure that you have the individual's attention. Standing in front of the person, making eye contact, touching

the individual, and using their name are all good ways of gaining and maintaining attention. Do not ask questions unless you are prepared to listen. Patience is important. Elderly individuals often take more time in retrieving information and assimilating data. Task performance is slower.

6. When communicating, attempt to eliminate environmental noise and disturbance. Sit down in a quiet place.

7. Simplify demands and questions. Use examples and images that the person can understand. Be concrete. Break tasks down into steps. Because of memory problems, an individual may not be able to make coffee alone; however, with help, cues, and step-by-step assistance, they may be able to complete the task. If this is too complicated and time consuming, folding napkins or sorting silverware might be suggested. Individuals with Alzheimer's need opportunities for success and a sense of accomplishment.

8. When receptive verbal abilities are impaired, use nonverbal ways of communicating. Demonstrate and illustrate. Pantomime may work.

9. Use repetition and multiple cues.

10. Consider the individual's emotional state. Individuals who are apathetic with low energy may respond to stimulation. Anxious or agitated sufferers from Alzheimer's need structure, stability, and a calm environment. Limit choices, the number of visitors at one time, and excitement.

11. Individuals in a state of catastrophic excitement do not respond to reasoning, thus making communication even more difficult. Methods of managing agitation and violence are discussed in Chapter 21. However, it is useful to attempt to anticipate situations and events which cause decompensation and eliminate them if possible. In cases of decompensation, remove the individual from the environment. Often, a direct command such as, "John, stop that," gains attention and will allow for removal from stimulation.

12. Communication through holding and touching often works when other methods do not. In making my assessments, I have discovered ways to reach and interact even with those in late-stage Alzheimer's.

Sara had not spoken or responded for two years. Following a neuropsychological assessment using very simple means such as tracking, counting, and asking her to say the alphabet, I took her hand. We sat in the quiet examining room for about ten minutes, and she held my hand and occasionally squeezed it.

Family can often reach the unreachable relative by giving love and being available to touch and hold. Listening to quiet music or singing an old familiar song might allow one to enter the unresponsive mute world of a loved one suffering from late-stage Alzheimer's. Then it might be time to say good-bye and allow staff to provide for the hygiene and medical needs of the vegetative but well-loved and remembered spouse, parent, or significant other.

CHAPTER 20

Treatment and Care:
General Principles

Ogden Nash writes about the elderly in his poem "Old Men." The theme of the poem is that society does not mourn old men or look at their death "with wonder" but that other "old men know when an old man dies."

Caretakers of the elderly have special problems and often ambivalent feelings. They wish to provide the best care but sometimes wonder why. Unconsciously, they may wish for death and relief and release not only for the loved one but also for themselves. Yet this thought produces feelings of guilt and often shame, especially when the elderly person is a beloved spouse or parent. These feelings are more intense when the elderly person is physically or emotionally ill. Caring for someone with Alzheimer's is not easy. This chapter focuses on general principles to help the caretaker.

Caring for the elderly requires recognition of the individual's special needs and limitations. This is especially true in the care of the elderly individual with Alzheimer's. The principles of recognizing limitations and defining the individual's needs is necessary when making plans for treatment and management, whether the individual be in a facility such as a hospital or nursing home or living with the family.

Identifying the nature and extent of disabilities and impairments requires a complete assessment. Alzheimer's patients can suffer from cognitive disabilities as well as physical and emotional problems. Often, the patient's physical or medical needs are identified but emotional needs remain untreated.

Chapters 12, 18, 28, and 29 discuss diagnostic procedures and treatment approaches for depression and anxiety. This chapter focuses primarily on cognitive impairment and special needs. Management of individuals with Alzheimer's is complicated because of problems with memory, impaired ability to learn new information, language disabilities, a tendency to be disorganized and disoriented, and personality changes.

Problems with memory means that the individual cannot carry out tasks that require more than one step because they cannot sequence. Problems with incremental learning leads to confusion and inability to adapt to new situations. Problems with language (both expressive and receptive) result in directions not understood and the individual being unable to communicate needs and feelings. Agitation and irritation often result. Personality changes can result in acting out. Aggressive or violent behaviors tend to take place as the disease progresses.

Disabilities and impairments vary depending on the stage of the disorder. Therefore, management and treatment plans must be upgraded to answer current needs, be they medical, emotional, or functional. During early-stage Alzheimer's, the individual is able to toilet and care for himself or herself more adequately than later in the progression of the disease. However, emotional needs tend to exist related to anxiety and confusion about one's situation. Caretakers must realize that the individual with early-stage Alzheimer's needs understanding, support, and reinforcement. During middle-stage Alzheimer's, the individual tends to be less depressed. With increased confusion and disorientation, there tends to be irritation and frustration with related anger. During this phase of the disease, the focus is on controlling acting out behaviors. During middle-stage Alzheimer's, there is also decreased functional ability with the need to help the individual with basic hygiene and body care tasks. Incontinence is common. During early- and middle-stage dementia, there is usually no particular increase in physical illness or disability, except in the case where there is a coexisting physical illness such as heart disease. However, as the disease progresses, systemic failures and emotional withdrawal tend to occur. During late-stage dementia, the focus turns to medical and health care. Cognitive and emotional processing shut down, with the individual becoming vegetative.

Families are often able to care for the individuals at home until the final stages of the disorder. However, as is discussed later, this is sometimes not possible or best for the individual. This chapter focuses primarily on how to care for the family member at home, although the principles apply for institutional settings as well.

The following case is that of a 75-year-old woman who had lived at home with her husband prior to entering a nursing home. She is suffering from delusional dementia and major depression. This case illustrates how the needs of the individual—as well as the abilities of the caretaker to provide for these needs at home—change, currently requiring more intensive help.

CASE #23: LILY

Lily had a history of emotional problems and psychiatric hospitalizations. Prior to the time of the assessment, her husband had been able to care for her at home. However, during the interview, he described her as "unmanageable." Her physical illnesses included hypertension, chronic heart failure, and arthritis. She was grossly overweight and needed help with ambulation. Her ability to function was further impaired by her cognitive problems. Memory was poor. She was not oriented and became confused and irritable. She was unable to perform tasks such as shopping and cleaning the house. The husband was responsible for her hygiene and basic health-care needs. However, she did not recognize the fact that she had cognitive problems and was unable to care for herself. Testing indicated that she was in early- to middle-stage Alzheimer's. It might have been possible for the husband to care for her at home for a longer period of time. However, her obesity and health problems created the need for more intensive care. Also, she had episodes of aggressiveness and violent acting out. She threatened her husband, threw objects at him, and destroyed personal property at home when angry. Her anger appeared to be related primarily to frustration, especially when limits were placed on her.

General principles regarding care—not only for this individual but also for others suffering from dementia—include using positive and negative reinforcement, use of distraction rather than confrontation, and reducing stimulation. Simplification and structuring will eliminate confusion and frustration.

The first step in developing a behavioral-management plan is to identify spared abilities and focus on these to provide the individual with Alzheimer's the greatest amount of autonomy and dignity. Individuals with Alzheimer's tend to become involved in issues of control with the caretaker. The fact that Lily insists on going home reflects her unrealistic assessment of her abilities. She cannot care for herself or make decisions about her own welfare; however, she did have the ability to recognize her family and her friends. Simple conversations were not difficult for her and did not cause anxiety. Thus, family and friends should be advised to continue contact. Lily also maintained the ability to complete rote tasks and seemed very pleased and happy when asked to fold napkins. She also was able to participate in church services at the nursing home.

She did become very anxious and irritated when there were changes in her environment. Individuals who have moved from their own home to a congregate care facility often feel threatened when someone encroaches on their territory or when there are changes in living situations. For this reason, consistency must be provided. This is true at home as well as in an institutional setting. Changing furniture arrangements or moving treasured objects can create catastrophic reactions. Caretakers are cautioned to be aware of this.

Structuring of time and activities is also important in dealing with Alzheimer's patients. Individuals with dementia are unable to plan and organize for themselves because of deficits in executive functioning; however, there continues to be a need for consistency. Alzheimer's patients are unable to plan their activities. While some individuals are content to perform rote tasks, others require activities to occupy their time. The need for time-consuming activities varies from individual to individual. Finding an activity for the individual is sometimes difficult; however, focusing on past interests and abilities often helps. The individual who used to enjoy travel is often satisfied looking at a travel magazine or book. On the other hand, some individuals tend to be restless or agitated most of the waking hours. Plans for physical activity must be made. Special situations and solutions are discussed in Chapter 21.

Decreasing the need to make decisions tends to reduce anxiety because individuals with Alzheimer's lack ability to make logical decisions. Activities should be planned based on the individual's level of functioning. The length of visits and the number of visitors should be limited. Activities should be changed to compensate for the loss of skills and abilities. In late-stage dementia, just holding hands and sitting listening to music might be of benefit. Asking questions, pushing the individual to perform beyond ability, and overstimulation result in increased anxiety, with the possibility of decompensation.

Often, family members overestimate the abilities and skills of the patient with Alzheimer's. Family parties may be considered a "special event"; however, the Alzheimer patient may not be able to comprehend or appreciate the event. This also emphasizes the importance of the family member or caretaker evaluating needs and functional level and changes as the disease progresses.

Initially, the individual may benefit from social activities and engagements. However, as abilities decrease, there is often the need for disengagement, simplification, and decreased stimulations. The need for stimulation varies depending on the individual's cognitive, functional, and physical condition and situation. One real problem facing the caretaker is how to provide physical activity and exercise. The ability for the individual to adjust to stimulation also tends to vary, with a decreased tolerance as the day goes on. This should be recognized when planning events and activities.

While individuals with Alzheimer's tend to have problems with cognitive abilities, positive and negative reinforcement can still be used by caretakers, especially during the early and middle stages. Behavior-modification techniques must be direct and simple. Cognitive methods such as reasoning will not be effective in cases of cognitive impairment. Praising behaviors such as going to the toilet tends to reinforce the behavior. Reminding the individual of this need is also useful. Mild reproachment can act as negative reinforcement. Again, it is necessary to accurately judge the level of ability and not make demands that exceed ability.

Environmental factors can affect the level of stress. Long-term care facilities have become more aware of this and are attempting to structure the environment for the benefit of the residents rather than strictly from a functional aspect. Many of the principles used by these facilities can be used by families to reduce stress in the home of individuals with Alzheimer's, since about four-fifths live at home. The purpose of environmental design in institutions should be to improve functional ability and the quality of life.

Simplifying the environment in these institutions as well as in the home tends to eliminate confusion and possible accidents. Removal of objects that are likely to fall or break is one way of reducing the risk of accident. Loose plugs and electric cords can create problems. Locks on doors and cabinets are practical in many situations. In nursing homes, residents who have a tendency to wander are fitted with alarm bracelets. Keys are used on elevators.

Special areas can be arranged in the home with items for the Alzheimer's patient, such as a table in the living room with activity items. Furniture should be safe and not easily moved. Edges should be rounded. Special care in regard to placement of furniture out of the flow of traffic is important when the individual has visual problems. Furniture should not be moved at random. Even the Alzheimer's patient's movements become habitual. Rocking chairs are often used to provide a form of exercise as well as relaxation.

Many nursing homes use gerichairs. These tend to have detrimental side effects, however, including deterioration in proprioceptive sense and muscle strength.

Soft music has been used effectively to reduce stress and promote calmness. Playing songs which were popular during the individual's more active and functional years has been used with good results. The elderly tend to suffer from hearing loss, so background music should be played at an appropriate level. Acoustics in the home or care facility should dampen extemporaneous noise. Unfortunately, many facilities use floor materials that are easy to clean without concern for sound levels. Television sets are also often allowed to blare. Residents with hearing problems might be provided with earphones for the television and radio or tape player. Beepers in hospitals and nursing homes also tend to be a source of irritation and distraction. Vibrating beepers could eliminate much of this distraction. The staff should be trained to be aware of sound levels and try to limit excessive noise.

Minimizing shadows, increasing the wattage of lightbulbs, providing diffuse sources of light, and limiting glare are all ways of increasing visual perspective and decreasing accidents. Removal of mirrors and use of night lights can reduce confusion.

Contrasting colors should be used for handrails, doorknobs, and stairs. Red and yellow are more easily seen than blues and greens. Strips of tape on the floor can be used to caution as well as to guide and direct the Alzheimer's patient. Symbols can be used rather than written words to identify areas in a institutional facility, such as a knife and fork for the dining room.

Allowing the individual with Alzheimer's to keep their own belongings and have some of their own furniture, whether moving in with family or in an intensive care facility, tends to reduce stress, although fear of loss of loved objects is common. A cabinet with an easy-to-use latch might be provided to store these items. During the day, the individual might be given their purse or a small bag to carry with them. Wheelchairs in nursing homes are commonly fitted with a small storage area or places where the resident can keep a few belongings.

Allowing for privacy as well as socialization is important in maintaining a level of dignity and self-respect. Knocking before entering the resident's room is not only polite but provides for a sense of control. Addressing the individual by their last name is also good form unless told otherwise. (In this book, first names have been used in case studies for reasons of simplicity.) In late-stage Alzheimer's, however, the individual may respond only to their first name because of memory problems and confusion.

Chapter 21 discusses specific management problems and solutions.

Chapter 21

Specific Management Problems and Solutions

In the poem, "Do Not Go Gentle into That Good Night," Dylan Thomas writes about the differing personal perspectives of individuals faced with death and, in particular, the emotions and behavior of his own father. Thomas suggests that one should not be passive in the face of death but rather "rage against the dying of the light." He continues that wise men, although they realize death must come, "do not go gentle into that good night." He also suggests that "good men," "wild men," and "grave men" rage against death. He then pleads that his father, too, "rage[s] against the dying of the light."

In developing a management plan for those suffering from Alzheimer's disease, it is important to recognize that many of the behavioral problems can be related to coexisting conditions such as depression and anxiety disorders and not just the cognitive impairments of dementia. One of the previous chapters discussed pharmacological treatment of agitation and anxiety as well as principles of psychotherapy.

In the poem prefacing this chapter, the wise, good, wild individuals going "into that good night" had reasons of their own to go with rage. This anger or rage was not related to the personality change of Alzheimer's but to personality characteristics. In dealing with Alzheimer's patients, we must recognize that some of the problems are related to the disease and some to preexisting factors. The individual who suffers from chronic depression will continue to be depressed in Alzheimer's. The individual who was demanding and controlling will probably become more demanding and controlling with illness, be that illness physical, emotional, or mental. Thus, the solutions to the "problem behaviors" discussed in this chapter vary from individual to individual and situation to situation. Family members probably already have developed some coping techniques and practices that they have used in the past. Distraction may work with one individual who becomes irritable and angry but may exacerbate these moods with another. The family should be aware of what responses have been effective in the past and incorporate them in a management strategy. The following suggestions or solutions are general in nature and based on the recognition that the Alzheimer's patient has problems with memory, adapting to new situations, impulse control, executive functions, and language.

The particular intervention or technique varies with the progressive nature of Alzheimer's. In the early stages, before reasoning and judgment abilities are severely impaired, it will be possible to identify a problem and discuss this with the sufferer. As the disease continues, behavior-modification techniques rather than cognitive approaches will have to be used. In late-stage Alzheimer's, behavior modifications will be of little value. However, as discussed previously, the individual will become more vegetative and management and care will be focused on health and sanitary needs rather than on behavior.

CASE #24: ARNOLD

According to his family, Arnold had always been angry. He was angry as a boy; angry as a father and as a husband; and now, at age 82, angry as an old man. During his middle-adult years, his anger resulted in the loss of job, alienation of his family, and lack of friends. His anger was expressed in episodes of rage and loss of control. It was usually focused with some one person as the object of his outburst. Now that he has Alzheimer's and is living in a nursing home, his rage is less specific. He tends to wander the halls cursing and muttering at staff members and other residents. When there is noise or confusion, he becomes more agitated and aggressive. This is the result of regression and an automatic response of the fight–flight syndrome. Reasoning with him does not reduce his agitation and combativeness. However, neuroleptic medication has reduced his oppositional and sometimes assaultive behavior to some extent. The staff has been instructed to watch for early signs of agitation and to remove him from the situation. He tends to become upset primarily prior to mealtimes. Also, one of the residents tends to cause him to become agitated and angry. This resident, who is not suffering from Alzheimer's, has been cautioned to stay away from Arnold or alert the staff in cases of escalation. Keeping the environment structured helps to some extent. The staff has also learned that calling the individual by his first name and saying, "Stop that," helps to distract him. Distraction is more effective than confrontation, although limits must be set and the safety of the other residents maintained.

Many patients suffering from dementia become very anxious and tend to "cling" to the caretaker. This is because they are confused or cannot provide for their own needs. They fear abandonment and desertion. Allowing these individuals to stay within sight of the caretaker eases anxiety but is not always possible, practical, or wise. Distraction with an activity sometimes provides temporary relief. Setting limits in a firm voice can be of benefit. Providing the individual with a caretaker possession such as a sweater may also work. During early-stage Alzheimer's, assurance of the patient's security is necessary because early-stage Alzheimer's patients tend to be more anxious than in later stages. During later stages, the patient is usually agitated with less focus. Restlessness, pacing, and fidgeting are common without explanation. Reassurance, attention, and affection can relieve this form of anxiety to some extent. As discussed earlier, antianxiety medication in the elderly patient tends to cloud sensorium and increase confusion and can cause paradoxical excitement.

Caretakers should attempt to provide a calm atmosphere and environment. Limiting stimulation is important. The mood of the caretaker is also important. Lashing out at the anxious Alzheimer's patient can cause a catastrophic response. Over a period of time, caretakers usually are able to discover how to distract the anxious individual and calm them. Staying calm, speaking in a soft voice, and setting the mood tend to be useful, although it is granted that the caretaker also has needs.

Dealing with abusive, demanding, and insulting remarks is another problem facing the caretaker. It is probable that these expressions reflect inner feelings of frustration and confusion and that accusing the caretaker of neglect, for example, is the patient's attempt to express this frustration. Alzheimer's patients seem to focus on one concern, such as going home or being taken advantage of by others. In effect, the individual is saying that things are not as they used to be. Often, accusations reflect feelings of loss, especially during early-stage Alzheimer's. There are also feelings of fear, and the accusations and demands are attempts to get attention and help. Ignoring insults and accusations or acknowledging the complaint simply is better than attempting to convince the Alzheimer's patient that they are wrong in the accusation. Realizing that individuals tend to lose impulse control and knowledge of social appropriateness might help. Explaining this to friends and neighbors on a need-to-know basis will help the caretaker avoid embarrassment. As society becomes more aware of the symptoms and nature of Alzheimer's, we should, most likely, become more sympathetic and understanding.

The individual who becomes combative presents real problems not only at home but also in an institutional setting. Removal from the situation causing the problem may have to be done physically. However, in general, it is best not to touch the individual because this creates increased threat. Use of restraints is covered by the mental code in most states. In the case of psychotic acting out, transfer to a mental hospital might be required to stabilize the individual and develop a management plan. The effect of psychotropic medication can then be observed and monitored. As discussed earlier, there is the possibility of an emotional illness, such as schizophrenia, coexisting with Alzheimer's disease. Delusional processes are also possible, related to a mental illness that is preexisting or coexisting. Recognizing what causes the combativeness is important, just as it is important to try and understand what creates anxiety in the Alzheimer's patient. Common causes include being pushed, asking the person to do or think about two things at one time, or asking the person to perform a task that the individual cannot accomplish. Again, it is important not to overestimate abilities and skills. New surroundings or different caretakers (nurses and nurses' aides included) can cause agitation, anxiety, or combativeness.

Not being listened to, understood, or attended to can cause acting out. Being tired or hungry increases the risk of behaving inappropriately. Early-stage Alzheimer's patients also tend to become upset when their sense of self or dignity is threatened. Specific situations such as being bathed may cause a reaction. Being patient, reinforcing appropriate behavior, and trying to understand and anticipate the individual's needs can improve behavior and lessen management problems.

Individuals suffering from Alzheimer's normally do not display symptoms of clinical depression, although during early-stage Alzheimer's, lethargy, sadness, and reactions to loss are common. As judgment and reality-conceptualization problems develop, specific losses are not as readily recalled; and the impact of the loss tends to diminish. An individual in middle-stage Alzheimer's may associate "home" with security and be preoccupied with "going home." This need can be answered by providing the individual with feelings of security. Continual reassurance may be necessary. Expressions such as "It's all right; I'll be here," and "I'll take care of you" often ease anxiety.

Where the individual is able to recall specific losses such as the death of a husband or the loss of a home, these issues can be addressed in therapy. Differentiating between clinical depression and sadness or anxiety which often accompany early Alzheimer's is important, however, in that depression can present as Alzheimer's. Diagnostic techniques are discussed in Part II.

Again, it is important to assess the individual's cognitive abilities when dealing with issues such as depression. It makes little sense to use cognitive therapy with a middle- to late-stage Alzheimer's patient, although the presenting problem may appear to be a loss or a grief situation.

Individuals with Alzheimer's do not usually consider suicide. During early stages, they may be angry, anxious, and confused. However, suicidal ideations are infrequent. Risk of suicide is diminished by the fact that executive functions are impaired, yet accidents and injuries are very common due to lack of judgment and common sense. The individual must be closely watched where there is risk, such as in the kitchen or bathroom. The environment should be modified to reduce risks by removing loose rugs and sharp objects.

Risk of falling is high among the elderly, especially those with Alzheimer's. Some medications have ataxic side effects. Weakness of bone and muscle, proprioceptive deficits, problems with awareness of environment, and visual problems exacerbate the risks. Medications should be checked for side effects. Guard rails on beds may be required. Gerichairs have been designed so that they are less restrictive and allow for some movement of muscles, although extensive use of these devices is not recommended during the initial stages of Alzheimer's. As Alzheimer's progresses, the individual will become less able to ambulate. Gait disturbances develop with increased risk of falling. However, keeping the person as active as possible tends to postpone muscle and health deterioration. Physical therapy should be considered for the bedridden patient. Turning the individual every two hours is necessary to prevent bed and pressure sores. The body must be kept clean and dry. Caring for the late-stage Alzheimer's patient at home might not be possible or practical.

During early- and middle-stage Alzheimer's, exercise is necessary not only for health reasons but also to help prevent agitation and improve sleep processes. Often, individuals with Alzheimer's remain physically able and relatively healthy long after cognitive and functional abilities have deteriorated. Regular exercise also tends to improve regularity. Walking around the house or nursing facility with the individual suffering from Alzheimer's is one way of exercising. Allowing the individual to hold your arm is better than holding on to them. In early-stage Alzheimer's, the individual can be taken shopping or to the mall. Pushing a grocery cart gives a sense of significance and can be used for a support. In nursing homes, individuals are often given a wheelchair to push rather than to sit. Supervised stair climbing can increase circulation. Going outside to walk with the individual provides variety and can improve sleep. Walking the same route eliminates disorientation and confusion.

Individuals with ambulation problems can exercise in a chair. Arm- and leg-raising movements are recommended. In early-stage

Alzheimer's, activities such as supervised gardening or water aerobics might be possible. Day-care centers often have exercise programs incorporated in activity schedules. When considering a more intensive care setting such as a nursing home, make sure that exercise, physical therapy, and occupational therapy are offered.

Exercise tends to improve sleep. Sleep–wake disturbance is very common among elderly patients with Alzheimer's. Nighttime wakefulness is the most frequent complaint. Individuals who are not kept active during the day tend to dose and then are restless at night. Pain at night also increases wakefulness. Managing sleep disturbance should begin by reducing sedating drugs, according to recent research. Analgesics, muscle relaxants, some neuroleptic drugs, and antianxiety medications tend to have the greatest sedating side effect. Maximizing out-of-bed time during the day and providing for some form of exercise is the second step. Stimulants such as coffee and tea can be used during the day but not with or after the evening meal. Bathroom needs should be attended to regularly, especially right before bedtime. A 9:00 P.M. bedtime is recommended, with some activity up until this time. Barbiturates are not recommended.

If the individual does awaken at night and wander, confronting them quietly and gently and putting them back to bed is the best approach. Leaving a night light on in the bedroom and bathroom reduces confusion. Soft music may improve sleep. Making sure that the bedroom is hazard free is very important.

The most common causes of death in individuals with Alzheimer's are pneumonia, dehydration, and malnutrition. Proper nutrition is necessary not only from a physical health aspect but also from a mental health standpoint. Individuals with dementia tend to forget to eat or lack the ability to plan and prepare proper and adequate meals. This is one reason that early-stage Alzheimer's patients need special care and supervision. Risk of injury is another reason.

During early-stage Alzheimer's, eating problems may develop because of emotional factors such as suspiciousness, paranoia, or change of living situation. Individuals who are moved to a nursing facility can be oppositional and defiant.

A proper diet, including plenty of fluids, is important. Often, water is not readily available or the individual forgets to ask. With age, problems with swallowing can develop. The patient with dementia may forget to chew or swallow. Providing the patient with soft foods can correct this problem. Nursing homes should be aware of problems with eating and provide the confused or demented individual with assistance. A liquid high-calorie diet is required in certain cases.

In some cases, the individual may no longer be able to eat or swallow. At this time, the family will have to decide whether to allow the insertion of a nasogastric tube, a gastro tube, or intravenous feeding. The aspects of this decision should be discussed with the physician. Ethical and legal issues, as well as medical issues, must also be considered.

As the person's dementia becomes more debilitating, problems with hygiene arise. Not only is the individual unable to care for himself or herself, but he or she may tend to resist help from others. Bathing the individual becomes a battle. This is especially difficult when the caretaker is the elderly spouse. Being aware of bathing and grooming habits in the past and adhering to these rituals is helpful in many cases. If the individual is accustomed to taking a bath, showering can cause anxiety and stress. Special appliances, such as a bath seat, can be purchased for the bath or shower to provide for safety. Fitting the tub or shower with railings is also suggested. Use little water in the tub and do not leave the individual alone. Eliminating the need to make a decision or decisions is also helpful. Alzheimer's patients should not be asked to choose a suit or dress, for example, from a wide selection of clothes. Asking to choose between even two items can result in confusion. Clothes that are easy to use such as sweatsuits and slip-on shoes are suggested. Clothes with snaps, velcro, and zippers are also better than clothes with buttons. Encouraging the individual to dress each morning and helping with grooming tends to improve the individual's sense of self and dignity. Complimenting the person on his or her appearance and encouraging him or her to look at himself or herself in the mirror can build self-esteem, especially in the early stages of Alzheimer's.

Individuals with Alzheimer's may behave in sexually inappropriate ways. This is primarily related to lack of judgment and impulse control. Confusion may lead to undressing in public or touching someone else or themselves in inappropriate ways. Masturbation may occur. These behaviors are related to forgetfulness rather than intending to shock or be offensive to others. Undressing can be controlled by using clothes which are difficult to remove such as a blouse with a zipper in the back or pants that are hard to unbutton.

Distraction is one way of dealing with inappropriate sexual behaviors. Often, individuals need to touch something. Providing them with an object to hold or carry provides a distraction as well as satisfies a need, similar to a child who carries or holds a doll. This may seem demeaning; however, management strategies that are effective and creative are often based on the realization that middle- and late-stage Alzheimer's patients have, indeed, regressed. Techniques in helping them as well as managing behavior must recognize that thought processes and cognitive abilities deteriorate to a very concrete and basic level, as do functional abilities.

Another issue that is often not addressed in the care and management of those with Alzheimer's is the issue of intimacy and sexuality with the spouse. (Sexual needs and issues are also not usually addressed in other cases, such as the institutionalized or residential care individual suffering from schizophrenia or mental retardation.) In many cases, a spouse cares for the individual with Alzheimer's. As the disease progresses, what once might have been an intimate and even romantic relationship deteriorates due to the inability of the Alzheimer's patient to respond in appropriate ways. Anxiety, anger, depression, and confusion during the early stage of Alzheimer's are very common. These responses interfere with a healthy and mutually rewarding relationship. The spouse also experiences emotional trauma and dysphoria. Personality changes and acting out, often associated with middle- to late-stage Alzheimer's, further impair intimacy. Little has been written or researched about this subject. However, it has been the experience of this clinician that continuing to provide love, attention, and nurturing is understood, accepted, and appreciated by the impaired partner. Gentle touching and holding seem to calm the agitated Alzheimer's patient. Although it may not be much, there are unspoken rewards for the spouse who knows in his or her heart that he or she has helped the loved one as he or she progress through the disease.

Another issue in managing Alzheimer's is the issue of social engagement versus disengagement. As discussed earlier, the stage of the disease, the individual's past social experiences and current level of social functioning, and personality traits and characteristics should all be considered. An individual who is avoidant should not be expected to become engaged as readily as someone with past social skills. Shy and self-conscious individuals might be encouraged to watch social activities from the sidelines. In a nursing facility, one-to-one comforting and assuring conversations with the staff are more beneficial than group activities.

As the disease progresses, activities must become less complicated. Day-care centers offer diversion and activity for the individual with early- to middle-stage Alzheimer's. Other community services are discussed in Chapter 24. In the case of institutionalization, the family should meet with the activity and social services staff to discuss past interests and skills and develop a plan to occupy the individual's time.

CHAPTER 22

Impact of Alzheimer's on the Family

CASE #25: CATHERINE

Catherine's husband died about fifteen years ago. At that time, Catherine was 60 years old. After the death of her husband, she continued living in the family home. She has two sons and a daughter who lived in the same town. The sons helped their mother with basic maintenance chores and the daughter and daughters-in-law visited three or four times per week. Recently, the family noticed that Mother was becoming more forgetful. On one occasion, one of the family members noticed a stove burner had been left on apparently overnight. Mother's house was becoming unkept. The garbage was not taken out regularly. This was unlike Mother in that she had been a meticulous housekeeper and efficient homemaker.

The family was also worried about Mother's eating habits and her ability to take her medications as prescribed. Mother's mood had also changed. She was becoming more withdrawn. She was aware of problems with memory and embarrassed about an inability to remember names and facts about her life and the family. Her response was to isolate herself. She had been very active socially. Now she stayed home and watched television.

Family concern led to a complete medical exam. No cause for her problems in memory and functional ability was found. A complete psychological assessment was recommended with the diagnosis of early-stage Alzheimer's. Her symptoms included problems with memory, orientation, deficits in social and independent functioning, denial, anxiety, and aphasia. She was able to follow directions and dress herself. At times, she had crying spells but was pleasant and able to relate to family members. She was not incontinent and had no physical disabilities.

The family was faced with the decision on how best to care for the needs of Mother at this time and how to plan for the future. As part of the assessment procedure, advice and counseling were provided (see Chapters 24 and 25 on care options). The family decided that Mother would live with one of the sons and his family. This decision was not easy. As in any family, there are priorities, time and availability constraints, financial considerations, and the needs of other family members to consider when making a decision on caring for an elderly parent. All three of Catherine's grown children had families of their own. The living arrangement decision for Mother was a difficult one and required professional help and advice to deal with unresolved issues from the past and emotional factors. The process was one of negotiation within the family. As Mother's condition and functional ability deteriorate, other choices will have to be considered. However, at this time, the family is able to provide for Mother's needs at home. Still, her illness had an impact on the family and required major adjustments, both financially and emotionally, and in living arrangements.

CASE #26: RUTH

Ruth was 74 years old when diagnosed as suffering from middle-stage Alzheimer's. Symptoms had appeared three or four years prior to the assessment. Before the disease, she had been socially and physically active. She was a community leader and served on the board of the local school. Her husband was also very involved, although he had retired about ten years earlier. He was 78 at the time of the assessment. Over the last two years, his physical and emotional health had begun to deteriorate because of his wife's condition. She required more and more help with basic tasks such as dressing and bathing. She also became easily frustrated and irritated. Her confusion and disorientation led to agitation and anxiety. Her husband attempted to calm her by reasoning with her. This only added to her agitation. At night, she wandered. The husband's sleep was disturbed, and he also became irritable. At times, he had problems with attention and concentration. In-home help was difficult to find and keep. The husband had little relief because the wife had become dependent on him as a small child can become dependent on a parent. When he left the room even for a few minutes, the wife began pacing and crying. The husband's physical condition became worse. Back pain developed because of the need to lift his wife. It was suggested that the husband and wife enter an intensive care facility. Initially, they shared the same room and bed; however, as the wife's condition deteriorated, she was transferred to an Alzheimer's unit on another floor. The husband continued to live in the facility so that he could visit her each morning and evening. He would go to her side each day and sit, holding her hand. The wife was mute, incontinent, and vegetative. She died six months later. The husband returned to his home. He died about six months after the death of his wife.

CASE #27: WILLIAM

William was a big man. He weighed over 250 pounds. He was 80 years old when assessed for Alzheimer's. He had a number of physical illnesses, including coronary artery disease, osteoarthritis, and chronic obstructive pulmonary disease. He was wheelchair bound. William and his wife lived in their own home until about two years ago when the wife died. William then went to live with a daughter. He had his own room yet required constant care. Family members stated that he had "never been a very happy person" and was demanding and irritable. With time, he became insulting to family members. He accused them of stealing his belongings and neglecting his needs. Memory problems began to develop. At times, he was disoriented and displayed signs of psychosis. The daughter had pledged to her mother that she would "never put Dad in a home." However, the father had become more and more difficult to manage, not only from a physical standpoint but also because of his emotional problems. His disruptive, aggressive behavior alienated his two adolescent grandchildren who lived at home. The daughter's husband was resentful about the time the daughter had to spend with the father as well as the deterioration in the marriage. The family was unable to take vacations. Father dominated the home and family life. The daughter began to feel guilty as well as angry. Her physical health deteriorated. Finally, it was decided to place the father in a nursing home. The father reacted by refusing to eat. At the home, he became violent and combative. The daughter began spending her entire day at the home to feed her father as well as to calm him. An assessment was ordered with the diagnosis major depression and senile dementia NOS (not otherwise specified) (mild to moderate). Medication and a behavioral-management plan were used in treatment. The family was advised to seek professional help to deal with feelings of guilt as well as unresolved family issues related to the experience of having "Dad" live with them for the last eighteen months.

Caring for family members with Alzheimer's disease is not easy and often has significant impact on all of the family members. Each family and each family member is affected differently depending on the relationship and level of responsibility for the individual with Alzheimer's.

However, denial, depression, anxiety, guilt, shame, and anger are common emotional responses among family members.

As individuals, we tend to resist change. Denial is an ego defense mechanism used to postpone the need to make change. This defense mechanism is used throughout life and allows us to gain time and eventually face reality in a more rational and reasonable manner. Marital problems are often denied in the hope that "things will get better." Alcoholism in the family is commonly denied not only by the individual who is dependent but also by other family members. Individuals tend to deny the symptoms of physical illness and thus postpone diagnosis and treatment. The same is true in the case of Alzheimer's. Denial is used in the hope that the symptoms are not, indeed, symptoms of Alzheimer's; and as discussed earlier, often they are not. However, family members tend to ignore or dismiss problems of memory, orientation, and cognition rather than seek professional help. (Seeking professional help is complicated by the fact that many individuals who present as being able and competent to diagnose Alzheimer's are not. The primary purpose of this book is to educate about the need for a complete and comprehensive assessment and the development of a treatment and management plan.)

Denial is common also because the development of Alzheimer's is progressive but not even. Individuals may have memory and orientation problems at night rather than during the morning. Psychosocial stressors and anxiety can exacerbate cognitive and functional abilities. Individuals in early-stage Alzheimer's tend to present as more capable and able because simple language skills are intact. Individuals with Alzheimer's also confabulate.

Family members may deny the existence of problems because of fear and lack of understanding. Accepting the fact that a loved one has Alzheimer's disease requires decisions about current and future care. These decisions can be difficult, especially because other family members become involved. Often, there are unresolved issues such as who provided care in the past or who was favored by the parent, elderly aunt, uncle, or grandparent. Legal and financial factors as well as availability must be considered. Denial that the loved one suffers from a progressive and debilitating disease postpones decisions about responsibility and care. However, an early and accurate diagnosis is essential.

Anger is another common response. Even in a good marriage, the prospect of caring for a spouse with dementia for a period of seven to ten years is frightening as well as disconcerting. Anger is often related to the "Why me?" syndrome. Role reversal causes anger. The adult child becomes the parent. The spouse becomes the mother or the father. The loved one becomes dependent, and the significant other becomes the caretaker. Families have their own problems. Adult children have been called the "sandwich" generation, with the need to care for their own children as well as their parents. The need to care for parents usually comes at a time when there are additional financial demands, such as college, as well as stress within the family system related to separation and emancipation of adolescent or young adult family members. Marital problems can also develop during this period. Caring for a parent with Alzheimer's adds to the stress of the family and has repercussions with each member. Teenage children often become the most angry and resentful.

The spouse who assumes the caretaker role has not only the responsibility and physical and financial demands to contend with but also the feelings of anger and depression that he or she has lost a partner for the later years of life. Loss of intimacy and sexual satisfaction exacerbate these feelings. Depression is common with other family members. An adult child may have lost a loving and available parent. Psychologically, we tend to have an image of security and safety while the parent lives, even if the parent may suffer from physical problems. With dementia, the opportunities for continued intellectual stimulation and rapport are gone. The hero is dead.

Chronic illness of any kind tends to cause anxiety in family members. This is especially true in the case of Alzheimer's disease. The caretaker becomes vigilant and alert to new and more severe signs of deterioration. Because the progression is patchy, there is not only hope but also disappointment. As the disorder progresses, care becomes more difficult and requires more time and energy. Anxiety over time creates the response of hopelessness and helplessness. The caretaker sees no end to the physical exhaustion and fatigue. They tend to become emotionally overwhelmed. This can lead to feelings of hatred, which lead to guilt and increased dysphoria. Ambivalent feelings such as "not doing enough" and hoping that "the end is near" are not uncommon. A confused emotional state results especially where there are unresolved relationship issues with the individual suffering from Alzheimer's. Individuals who have grown up in a dysfunctional family tend to have problems throughout the life course. These problems become more apparent with the disability or dependency of the significant individual later in life, especially in cases of role reversal. Some studies suggest that abuse of the elderly is related to earlier relationship problems that have not been identified and addressed.

Because middle- and late-stage Alzheimer's patients tend to develop behavior problems, there is more likelihood of mistreatment due to frustration, fatigue, and emotional overload of the caretaker. This can lead to guilt and shame.

Shame can also be related to caretaker feelings of embarrassment due to inappropriate actions and behavior of the family member with Alzheimer's. Inability to control body functions, aggressive behavior, and such acts as undressing or touching oneself or others inappropriately are common in middle- and late-stage Alzheimer's. With Alzheimer's, as with other mental illnesses in the family, it is not uncommon for other members to feel a sense of shame.

It must be realized that Alzheimer's disease is an organic disorder. It is not caused by environmental conditions. Family members are not responsible for the illness. Chapter 23 discusses how the caretaker can cope with Alzheimer's in the family not only from an emotional approach but also from a practical approach. Chapters 19 and 21 have discussed communication and management techniques.

CHAPTER 23

Advice for Family Members

It has been estimated that 2.5 to 4 million Americans suffer from Alzheimer's. The probability that a loved one, significant other, or member of one's extended family will develop the disease has become greater with the aging of America. This chapter is devoted to techniques to deal with one's feelings, emotions, and situation when a family member develops the disease. Recommendations are listed in the remainder of this chapter.

1. Education. It is most important that the family member become familiar with the disorder, including the prevalence, the symptoms, the course, and how to help the individual who is suffering from the disorder. Education is the operative word. Learning about the disorder allows one to react in a rational and adaptive way as well as make plans for the future. Alzheimer's disease is a progressive organic disorder that is too often misdiagnosed, mistreated, and mismanaged. Knowing that there are reversible forms of dementia will aid the family member and should result in the demand for a comprehensive and complete assessment.

2. Make arrangements for an assessment. This assessment should include inquiry to family and medical history; a clinical interview with the individual suspected of suffering from Alzheimer's; an evaluation of intellectual, psychological, cognitive, and functional abilities; and the development and implementation of a treatment or management plan. Anything less than this is likely to result in misdiagnosis and mismanagement.

The family should insist that the assessment be made by an individual who is interested, patient, knowledgeable, and competent. Knowledge of and training in the field of geriatric medicine or psychology is vital. Follow-through to implement the management is also vital. Too often a diagnosis of Alzheimer's is given after a brief interview with the family, patient, or both, and a five-minute mini mental status exam. Often, the diagnosis is inaccurate. To compound the travesty, the family and subject are often left with no direction or guidance. Hopefully, this book will provide family members with information vital in coping with Alzheimer's in the family.

Knowing about the nature, course, treatment, and management of Alzheimer's is not sufficient to diagnose the disorder. Family members are advised not to attempt to diagnose the disorder from observed symptoms. Family members should seek immediate professional help. Facilities with complete diagnostic and management services are available in most areas of the country. The services of a physician to supervise medication, if necessary; a psychologist to assess the patient and make management recommendations, as well as provide psychotherapy for the patient and the family; and a social worker to determine functional and independent living abilities, as well as provide linkage for community services, are probably desirable.

3. *Involve the entire family in decisions concerning care and management.*   It is important that family members discuss their feelings and emotions as well as identify their willingness to become involved in and responsible for various aspects of the care and management. Financial aspects should be discussed. Expectations should be made explicit, and negotiations should be honest and direct. It is best to be as specific as possible. In this way, misunderstanding will be avoided. Plans for the future should also be discussed. Responsibilities and caretaker tasks and assignments will probably change over time. It might be of benefit to assign one family or family member to research what community services are available (see Chapter 24). In the case of Alzheimer's disease, the family must be realistic that there will be the necessity for more intensive care.

Planning for family involvement and deciding on responsibilities and caretaker task performance may require the assistance of a professional not only to help the family determine what services are available but also to help the family deal with emotional and interpersonal issues. The agency that provided the assessment should be available for such services. Insurance usually covers part of the costs of family therapy as well as individual therapy. The individual who is suffering from Alzheimer's should be included in the planning processes as much as possible. The degree of involvement will depend not only on the individual's cognitive and mental abilities but also on personality factors and interpersonal issues in the family system. Professional help might be required at this time to help the individual with early-stage Alzheimer's understand and accept the need for care. In the event of coexisting mental or emotional illness, pharmacological and psycho-therapy strategies must be developed (see Chapters 17 and 18).

4. Consider joining a support group. Support groups provide education and association with other individuals facing similar situations and problems. There is often relief in knowing that one is not alone and that there are sympathetic individuals available to provide support, comfort, and advice. Venting one's feelings of guilt, anger, depression, and anxiety and realizing that others are experiencing similar feelings can be therapeutic.

5. Consider individual therapy if the symptoms of depression, anxiety, hopelessness, helplessness, and anger become overwhelming. Venting is not always enough. As suggested in Chapter 22, the illness of a loved one—whether physical or emotional—can be traumatic. Repressing feelings related to a traumatic situation is not emotionally healthy or wise.

6. Be aware of how the illness of the family member affects the other members and how it affects your role, relationship, and behavior within your own family. In the case of an elderly spouse with Alzheimer's, do you as the caretaker avoid family celebrations and get-togethers? Have you become isolated, withdrawn, angry, and depressed? As the adult child of a parent with Alzheimer's, do you focus on the parent's needs and ignore the needs of your own family? Re-evaluate your own feelings, behaviors, and priorities. You as a family member cannot reverse the course of Alzheimer's. You also cannot care for an individual in late-stage Alzheimer's without extensive help. Recognizing one's limitations is a part of successfully letting go. As discussed, spending every day with an Alzheimer's patient in a nursing home or intensive-care facility is not always desirable. It keeps the individual dependent and does not allow for participation or involvement in activities which might be therapeutic or desirable. In early-stage Alzheimer's, involvement in physical, occupational, and activity therapy is usually beneficial for the patient.

7. Loving detachment. There will come a time when the individual with Alzheimer's will not recognize you and eventually will not respond. This does not mean that you must physically leave the individual. Such activities as touching, holding, listening to music, or just sitting in the same room are sometimes calming and therapeutic, not only for the family member with Alzheimer's but also for the caretaker. However, there will come a time to say good-bye and realize that the spirit has left. At that time, tears often help. When the time comes, you must say good-bye—at least emotionally—and go on with your life.

8. Outside involvement and the development of interests other than those related to the loved one with Alzheimer's are vital. This may appear to be obvious; however, very often the caretaker has drifted into a situation of codependency driven by guilt and anxiety. Just as mothers need mother's morning out, away from the responsibility and constant care of an infant, you need time away. In some ways, Alzheimer's patients are like infants, especially in late-stage Alzheimer's. You must make arrangements for relief. In early Alzheimer's, day-care centers are often beneficial. Make plans for the future as the disease progresses.

9. Develop a stress management plan.   Relaxation, diet, and exercise are important.

10. Rid yourself of guilt.   Share the responsibility of caretaking. Realize that eventually you will need professional help.

11. Begin dealing with your feelings of grief and loss.   This is part of the processes of healthy emotional detachment. Where the relationship has been one of love and closeness, there will be grief and feelings of emptiness. However, because the individual with Alzheimer's usually lives for seven to ten years after the disease has been diagnosed, there is not always a specific time to deal directly with the loss of one who used to be vital, alert, loving, and aware. Also, the process of closure is impeded by one's involvement in care. However, near the end of the disease, you as the family member will have to deal with your grief. Coping with resentments and feelings of anger is also necessary and important.

Including other family members is often helpful. Review the good times. Look at pictures, videos, and films of family events and affairs. Review how the individual touched you and enriched your life. Allow other family members to do this also.

12. Finally, do all you can and then have faith.   Remember the twelve-step motto, "One day at a time." After the loved one has died, you may want to become involved in helping others deal with similar situations. Serving as a volunteer might ease your pain. Or you may want to go on a long trip. Whatever you decide, be assured that your love, involvement, and caring have not been wasted. You have done your best to ease another's pain and suffering.

CHAPTER 24

Utilizing Community Services and Resources

If I had known I was going to live this long, I would have taken better care of myself.
—Comment from an 87-year-old man during an assessment

Growing old ain't for sissys.
—Paul Newman

The aging process varies among individuals. Physical, emotional, and cognitive skills, abilities, resources, and capacities differ among same-age cohorts, as illustrated by the case studies in this book. An individual may be alert, functional, and autonomous well into his or her 80s, while another may be disabled and impaired at an early age. Physical, emotional, and cognitive disabilities result in the need for assistance in living and functioning. Obviously, the type of assistance depends on many factors. Inability to care for one's needs because of medical and physical problems is the most common reason for entering an extended-care facility. However, emotional and cognitive problems can also be causal factors. The cases presented illustrate how physical, emotional, characterological, and mental condition factors relate.

An individual who suffers a stroke or is incapacitated because of late-stage osteoarthritis can become depressed, anxious, and angry. Often, there is a tendency to give up. Feelings of hopelessness and helplessness can develop. An individual who was able to care for himself or herself before a stroke may become despondent over the loss of functional and physical abilities and resist rehabilitation therapy.

Incontinence often develops in the elderly because of problems with muscular control. This condition tends to be a narcissistic insult with associated feelings of shame and depression. In-home care becomes more difficult when the individual is incontinent.

Early-stage Alzheimer's patients may benefit from in-home care; however, there is often the need for more extensive professional help as the disease progresses. A great deal of progress has been made in the last twenty years in providing in-home care services for the elderly, not only those living independently but also those living with their families. Services have been provided by the public sector as well as the private sector. In fact, one of the greatest growth industries is that of providing in-home care services for the elderly and other groups of individuals with disabilities and functional incapacities.

Third-party providers appear to have realized that, from a financial standpoint, it is beneficial to provide care in the least expensive but also the least restrictive setting.

Hospital stays following a medical procedure have been reduced. Many operations are performed on an outpatient basis. The same is true with the provision of psychological services. Until about 1990, for example, the standard treatment for drug addiction was hospital treatment for four to six weeks. Now psychiatric hospital facilities are used for detoxification. Intensive outpatient treatment programs have replaced the four- to six-week inpatient programs. The same is true in treating other forms of mental illness.

The provision of psychological services, including psychological and neuropsychological testing and assessment is commonly done on an outpatient basis. In some cases, the psychometrician or neuropsychologist will come to the home of an individual suspected of suffering from a mental illness, including Alzheimer's. This offers a number of advantages. The patient tends to be less anxious and upset. The home environment can be observed as well as how the individual functions and carries out various health-care tasks. Family members can be interviewed and a social history taken.

Other services that can be provided in-home include cleaning services, physical and occupational therapy, nursing services, and such things as meal preparation and shopping. Many of these services are covered as Medicare and health-care benefits.

This chapter discusses utilizing various community-based services. Chapter 25 focuses on institutional placement and intensive-care issues, as opposed to community services.

The coordination of services for an elderly patient is a time-consuming and complicated task and often requires professional help. One reason that a complete assessment including functional abilities and needs is suggested is to develop a treatment plan. While it is the family's task to make decisions in regard to specific need and service requirements, social workers and caseworkers tend to have the information available regarding service and contact–contract methods.

Case managers have been a part of community service systems for some time. Now, with the aging of America, caseworkers are becoming more involved with the elderly. Geriatric case managers are often helpful in preventing unnecessary admission to a nursing home. The provision of in-home services can postpone the need for institutionalization in cases of early-stage Alzheimer's.

One of the best sources regarding available resources for individuals suffering from dementia is The Alzheimer's Disease and Related Disorders Association, otherwise known as the Alzheimer's Association. This is a privately funded volunteer organization. Local chapters can be located by contacting the national headquarters, located at 919 North Michigan Avenue, Suite 1000, Chicago, IL 60611–1676, or by calling 800–621–0379. Some of the local chapters have resource centers. They usually provide education and support services.

The National Stroke Association (NSA) is a nonprofit organization with the goal of educating the public, stroke victims, and their families about the impact of a stroke on the individual. The contact number for the NSA is 303–762–9922.

Many other national organizations have state and local chapters, which can provide information on available resources. The Area Agency on Aging and the Aging Information Office (AIO) link senior citizens with community resources. While the Agency is not directly involved with services for individuals with Alzheimer's, the information will provide sufferers and their families with resource data. Lists of senior day-care centers, nursing homes, and transportation services are available.

Investigating the availability of various services and costs on the local level is a time-consuming job because no one agency normally coordinates and provides the services. Contacting state, county, and local service providers is often necessary on a one-to-one basis. Often, individuals with physical, emotional, and cognitive problems need many different types of services. Some programs provide services such as dental care, eye examinations, legal services, prescription medication at reduced cost, and transportation. Meals on Wheels provides hot meals for those who cannot leave home. Nutritional counseling and shopping is provided by some agencies, as well as chore services and other homemaker services. Home health care and personal care aides will help in bathing and other basic needs in the home.

Because many families prefer to keep the individual who is suffering from dementia at home as long as possible, the demand for in-home services has greatly increased. The cost of these services is often prohibitive, however. In general, registered nurse care services on a physician's order are covered by Medicare and other insurance providers.

Day care for individuals with dementia is becoming more readily available. Adult day-care programs commonly offer from several hours to most of the day of structured care in a group setting. A hot meal, exercise, and activity programs such as crafts, music, and art are components of a well-developed program. Most of these programs are during the daytime hours and only on weekdays. Often, the client population is mixed with clients suffering from physical as well as emotional or mental problems. Patients with acting out or behavioral problems are usually not accepted. However, an increasing number of facilities have been developed to provide custodial care for those individuals with limited cognitive abilities. The goal of day-care facilities is to improve the quality of life for the individual client as well as relief for the caretaker.

Services available as well as quality of care vary from facility to facility. Before making a decision about day-care placement, it is wise to review the needs of the individual with Alzheimer's as well as the individual's abilities and disabilities. Some individuals will benefit from social stimulation; others will not. Some may benefit from activity therapy; yet others will become agitated, frustrated, and anxious. It is important for the staff members to be aware of the needs and likely responses of the family member suffering from Alzheimer's and to develop a program to answer these needs. Some individuals who are suffering from dementia will not be able to adjust to day-care living. While day-care services are commonly less expensive than in-home services, insurance usually does not cover the cost.

Respite care is another option, which may be covered by Medicare. Respite care is short-term inpatient or outpatient care intended to provide the primary caretaker with temporary relief from care responsibilities and duties. Care can be provided in a nursing home, foster home, boarding home, or other facility, usually for a weekend or even a week. Medicare limits coverage to eighty hours per year, which, while often not enough, does reflect the growing awareness on the part of government that older adults and their families do suffer from non-medical problems and may require assistance. This type of assistance, however, might result in separation anxiety; and the short-term relief might not be worth the effort required to make the arrangements. In the case of respite care, it is suggested that the facility be visited to assure that the family loved one is cared for in a kind and appropriate manner.

Recently, the number of group homes (as opposed to nursing homes) has increased. These facilities are usually around-the-clock care centers. These homes are regulated by various state and local agencies. Again, the type and level of care must be investigated. Cost for this type of facility is normally more than that for day care but less than that for nursing home care.

Companionship care at home has also increased in availability. Home health-care aides and companions provided by private agencies are usually more expensive than those contracted for on a direct basis. However, a family member usually will spend a great deal of time locating a companion and may not be able to judge the individual's abilities and character. The results can be unpredictable. When hiring an in-home companion, family members should not expect the companion to be a housekeeper. Preparing meals, companionship, and possibly such services as helping the individual bathe is about all that can be and should be expected. Discussing and negotiating fees, services, and schedules should be done before an agreement is made.

Referral by an agency does not guarantee satisfaction. It is up to the family member (hopefully with the help or assistance of a caseworker) to make the decisions regarding the level of care needed and how and where to contract for these services. In-home service workers should be bonded. Those who care for individuals with dementia should have some training. Certification of aides and caregivers is sometimes required. Check into the provider's background and experience. In the case of the health-care provider working for an agency, experience and training can be more easily ascertained. However, continued monitoring of the level and quality of services needed and provided is recommended. Alzheimer's is a progressively debilitating disease, and family members will be required to be aware of changes in abilities—both functional and cognitive—and needs.

Alzheimer's disease is considered to be a "custodial" disorder, which is not covered by Medicare, Medicaid, or, in most cases, private insurance. Medicare is a program to pay for acute care, not a chronic disorder such as Alzheimer's. However, Medicare will provide for up to 150 days of rehabilitation or nursing care service for those with medical illnesses. Dementia is not considered to require nursing home services; however, an individual with Alzheimer's often suffers from a physical or medical illness that does require treatment and care. There is no longer the requirement that the individual enter directly from a hospital. Caseworkers, as well as personnel at various facilities, will be able to help the family in determining costs and eligibility for services. Medicare coverage information can be obtained through a local Social Security office.

Medicaid is a federal government program administered by the individual states. Information on benefits can be obtained through local human services offices. Qualification for benefits depends on the amount of income and assets owned by the individual. In general, individuals are required to have spent their own assets before Medicaid will pay for benefits. About two-thirds of all residents living in nursing homes are covered by Medicaid. Nursing home care is expensive. This is one reason that less costly alternatives are being developed to care for the elderly. Unfortunately, policymakers have been slow to realize the cost advantages of providing services in the least restrictive setting.

Eligibility for Medicaid benefits as well as specific services covered varies from state to state. Coverage and benefits tend to change from time to time. Consulting an attorney with specific knowledge regarding Medicaid law might be of some benefit when confronted with the need for intensive or institutional care.

This leads us to Chapter 25. Eventually, nursing home or other institutionalized care will probably be needed for the individual suffering from Alzheimer's. Chapter 25 addresses issues related to finding a nursing home or other intensive-care facility.

CHAPTER 25

Choosing a Congregate Care or Nursing Home Facility

The need for special care and services, as well as the acceptance of this need, varies from individual to individual and situation to situation. The majority of the elderly live independent, autonomous lives, especially in cases where there are no serious illnesses, injuries, or cognitive problems. Individuals in early-stage Alzheimer's are often able to function in a relatively autonomous and functional manner with the help of family and friends, especially when community support services are available. Some of these services have already been discussed. They include the following:

Community care services
Home response systems
Home health care
Companion services
Respite care
Day care

With these support services, the elderly are often able to live independently or with family. However, with aging there is not only the possibility for the need for more intensive, around-the-clock services and care but also the desire. In Chapters 20 and 21, the disengagement versus engagement theory was discussed. Others resist giving up their homes, their sense of independence, and their autonomy. Adjustment to group living is difficult. An example of this is Mary. While Mary is not suffering from Alzheimer's, many of her responses—including confusion, anxiety, and resistance to help—are similar to those of individuals in early- or middle-stage Alzheimer's who have been moved from a less restrictive living situation to an institutional setting.

CASE #28: MARY

Mary was 86 years old when she was encouraged by family members to move into a group care home. Mary's husband had died about six months before the move. According to the family, the husband, who was three years older than his wife, took almost complete charge of the house and housekeeping operations. The couple had a variety of in-home services provided through the community and county.

The family stated that Mary was very passive, dependent, and unable to make decisions regarding the home and her own life. An assessment resulted in the diagnoses of major depression (recurrent severe), generalized anxiety disorder, and somatization disorder. The individual was able to function in a fairly adequate manner with the help of her husband; however, it was determined that her ability to do so at the time of the assessment was greatly diminished following the death of her husband.

Although it was decided that group living was the best alternative (in part, because of the unavailability of family and unwillingness to provide a home for the 86-year-old widow), the adjustment was not smooth. This was, in part, because of grief and the loss of the husband. (Recommendations to alleviate depression were made.) However, it was also because the individual suffered from chronic depression and anxiety. Her response to placement was to focus on her medical problems. Her complaints were constant and continual. She was unable to relate to peers and refused social involvement. Focusing on her physical problems was a way of avoiding dealing with her anxiety and loss as well as fears about the future. It also was an attempt to obtain attention.

Change is difficult for individuals suffering from Alzheimer's disease—just as it was for Mary—and for many of the same reasons. Mary had grown dependent on her husband for her needs. As cognitive and functional abilities deteriorate in cases of Alzheimer's, the individual becomes less functional and more dependent. Because they are confused and disoriented, they feel threatened. Because they cannot make their needs known (or do not know what they need), they often become angry and agitated. Any change can result in decompensation. The move to a group home or setting results in a change in environment, caretakers, and living situation. However, the decision to move a loved one to such a facility is necessary, often because of the inability of the family to provide the needed care.

The previous discussion has focused on situations where the individual has lived independently or with family, and the need arises for placement in a nursing home or similar facility. In situations like this, family members must make the decision for transfer to a more intensive care facility.

Another arrangement, called continuing-care retirement—as opposed to living independently or with family—has become an option. In many cases, however, because of the expense, this option is available only to those who are financially independent. Individuals with Alzheimer's are not usually considered by continuing-care retirement communities. However, in some cases where the spouse is functional, arrangements can be made.

The standard procedure in a continuing-care or life-care arrangement is to move initially into an apartment. The individual is provided with some services such as security check. Usually, residents can eat in their own apartments or eat some of the meals in a group dining room. This is true in a congregate housing facility. However, in congregate housing, linkage is usually not provided with medical or nursing home facilities.

The resident of a life-care facility is guaranteed continued care even as needs increase. As the need for care does increase, the individual is transferred to an assisted-care unit or wing where staff members provide such services as bathing and meal preparation. Eventually, the resident may need nursing home services, in which case, another transfer is made within the system.

Costs for continuing care include an entry fee (starting at $15,000) as well as monthly charges. These charges range from $150 to $3,000 per month. Because of the initial entry fee and commitment for life, it is recommended that the individual considering such a move (or the family) make sure that the services and physical facilities meet one's needs. The advice of an attorney might be considered. Information on accreditation can be obtained from the Continuing-Care Accreditation Commission (202–783–2242).

The decision to enter a continuing-care retirement facility comes before physical, emotional, or cognitive disability. Often, family members are faced with the sudden need of placing a loved one who has been cared for by the family but requires more intensive care in a nursing home. Once this decision has been made, the family is faced with the dilemma of choosing a facility. The following paragraphs are directed to helping the family make this decision.

Advice from knowledgeable professionals is often available. As part of an assessment for Alzheimer's, a treatment and management plan should be developed. The plan should include advice on various facilities and services available. This advice should be based on the needs of the individual. Information on the impairments and disabilities as well as resources comes from a complete evaluation of physical, functional, emotional, and cognitive abilities, as discussed in Chapters 22 to 25. Advice might be that the individual can continue at home with certain in-home services provided or that the individual needs residential services.

Lists of nursing homes are available from various sources, including the Alzheimer's Association, Area Agency on Aging, state and local health departments, and state accreditation agencies. All nursing homes provide personal care and residential services, including room and board and various activities; however, the range of services and level of care varies. Skilled nursing facilities (SNFs) provide around-the-clock nursing for convalescent as well as chronically ill patients. Registered nurses (RNs), licensed practical nurses (LPNs), and nurse aides provide the care. Physical and occupational therapy is usually offered.

Personal care facilities do not require highly trained or licensed personnel. Services include assistance with bathing, dressing, eating, and ambulation. Where medical problems are not primary, personal care facilities may be sufficient for individuals with dementia. However, Medicare usually does not provide coverage for personal care. In the event that the individual with Alzheimer's needs medical as well as personal care, a nursing home appears to be the best choice.

The first step in choosing a nursing home is to make an appointment with the administrator or admissions department and arrangements to visit the facility. Also, discuss funding possibilities and financial arrangements. Financial arrangements should be in writing and include initial and ongoing costs and expenses. Obtain a list of extra charges and inquire how the resident's personal funds are handled. Also inquire if there is a rebate for time spent at home on visits.

More than one visit to the facility is suggested before a decision is made. An unannounced visit is suggested. During the visits, one should observe the level of care, cleanliness, and safety. A smell of urine suggests inadequate care. Ask about activity and physical and occupational therapy. Discuss levels of care, especially if there are special facilities for Alzheimer's patients. Inquire about medication and behavior-management strategies. Is there a social services department? Are counselors or therapists available? Is there a family support system? What medical services and linkages are available? Are the surroundings pleasant and well lighted? Are single rooms available, and at what cost? Are personal possessions and furnishings allowed? Are children allowed to visit? How are the resident's privacy and personal belongings protected? What is the level of training and certification of the care providers? Make sure the home and the administrator are licensed and fire and safety regulation compliance is certified. Is the facility convenient for visiting? Talk to the head nurse and staff about the facility, their experience, and their experiences in caring for the elderly, especially an elderly patient with dementia.

Most staff members are truly dedicated. Their job is not easy. Ask the staff about training seminars and educational lectures provided, such as "how to communicate with patients with dementia" or "dealing with the aggressive, violent patient." Ask them if they have read this book or other books on Alzheimer's.

Talk to the activity director. What type of exercise is provided, especially for those suffering from Alzheimer's? Who supervises activities and exercise? Are most of the residents in wheelchairs or geriatric chairs and, if so, why? What social activities are provided? Ask to see the policy regarding use of restraints. How often is the use of psychotropic drugs reviewed? Is a neuropsychologist available for consultation? Do the consulting physicians have experience in geriatric medicine? How is incontinence managed?

How are patients' rights protected? What is the policy regarding life-sustaining measures? How is the food? Visit during mealtime to observe the level and type of care, as well as the quality of the food. What is the policy regarding use of nasogastric tubes or other feeding devices?

Recently, nursing homes have recognized the special needs of residents who are suffering from both medical problems and Alzheimer's. The Alzheimer's Association will provide information on the location of these facilities. When considering placement in such a facility, questions such as cost, levels of care, and special services should be discussed. Again, a number of visits to the unit is recommended.

Another recent trend in the care of individuals with Alzheimer's is the construction of home-like facilities. One of the first such facilities is the Wealshire in the Chicago area. The developer of this project stresses the importance of moving away from the medical model, although medical services will be available. Each household of sixteen to twenty-two individuals will have a kitchen, living and dining rooms, laundry, and yard. Involvement in daily living tasks will be stressed, including gardening, laundry, and setting and cleaning the table. The emphasis is on feeling useful, feeling secure, and feeling loved. While living in a setting such as this will not delay the progress of Alzheimer's, it does improve quality of life and provide the family with a sense that a loved one is being cared for. Day care and respite care are also scheduled to be available. This care is not inexpensive, however.

In the future, it is hoped that facilities will become available at reasonable costs to care for the needs of a loved one with Alzheimer's.

CHAPTER 26

Ethical and Legal Issues

This chapter focuses on ethical, moral, and legal issues in the diagnosis and treatment of Alzheimer's as well as in the area of patient rights and family involvement. Caretakers, medical and mental health providers, and care facilities are licensed by state and federal law. Each state has different requirements for certification and licensing. Individuals who provide services must operate within the boundaries set by law. Physicians may prescribe medication and treat physical illnesses; however, in most cases, they are not trained to administer and interpret neuropsychological or psychological tests. In fact, some states restrict the use of these instruments to licensed psychologists. Psychologists are not allowed to prescribe medication, with the exception that some states do allow prescription of psychotropic drugs with special training. Psychologists diagnose and treat primarily mental illnesses and emotional problems. The use of psychotherapy is restricted by some states, allowing only licensed individuals to practice. However, there are a number of unlicensed and uncertified practitioners who call themselves therapists or counselors.

The practice of nursing is regulated by each state. Social workers are also licensed or certified. Social workers were trained initially to offer linkage between the client and the community and provide social services. More recently, they have become involved in such areas as group counseling and family therapy.

It is unethical as well as illegal for a health-care provider to perform or provide services beyond his or her area of training and ability. This is one reason that a multidisciplinary approach is recommended in the diagnosis, treatment, and management of the dementias. However, competition often develops with legal battles regarding rights and privileges between the professions.

Fortunately, there are legal restrictions to providing service beyond one's level of competency and training, as outlined in licensing and certification law. Also, each profession is responsible for policing its own members; and complaints can be addressed to state professional associations and licensing boards.

Ethical and legal issues are also to be considered in relation to confidentiality and disclosure. State law provides for confidentiality between patient and physician, client and attorney, parishioner and clergy, and psychologist and client. Questions and problems related to confidentiality can arise. For example, under law, a psychologist has the duty to warn an individual whose life has been threatened by a patient, even though this information is given during a confidential therapeutic session. If a patient threatens suicide, the physician or therapist is required to take action to prevent suicide. This can include notifying the police and having the individual hospitalized for an evaluation of risk.

Professionals who diagnose and treat the elderly have problems related to need to know and confidentiality. Often, a diagnostician is called upon to judge the abilities of an individual related to the possible need for treatment in an institutional facility such as a nursing home. The arrangements for such an assessment are usually made by the family. The question arises regarding the obligation of the diagnostician to keep the information confidential.

If the elderly subject is under guardianship, confidentiality is not an issue. This is true in situations where there is a court order for an assessment to judge competence. In the case of the risk of suicide, information can be disclosed and steps taken for hospitalization. However, ethical as well as legal issues arise in situations where the individual is not under guardianship and expresses a desire for information, including information which might be related to ability to care for self, competence, or the need to be placed in a nursing home, not to be disclosed. There is also the issue of patient rights and an individual's resistance to placement in a nursing home. The following cases illustrate the wide range of attitude not only about placement in a group living situation but also views of life and death. Should an individual who expresses the desire to die be encouraged to live? What are the ethical and moral obligations of the physician, the therapist, the social worker, the staff, and the family? Sue wants to die.

CASE #29: SUE

Sue is an 88-year-old woman who entered a nursing home about 2.5 years before she was assessed. Prior to entering the nursing home, she had lived with a daughter. She entered the nursing home following the fracture of a hip. Her chart indicated that she suffered from glaucoma, osteoporosis, and arthritis. Auditory ability was severely impaired. She was unable to walk and thus was confined to a wheelchair. She was unable to dress or bathe herself and had to be assisted when eating because of problems with vision and fine motor ability.

Initially, on admission to the home, she had been involved in social activities and events. However, within the last three months, she had become isolative and withdrawn. Mental abilities were intact; however, interaction with others was becoming more difficult because of vision and auditory problems. It was determined that these problems could not be corrected.

Sue had lived a rich and full life. She had raised a family and was involved in her community. Until her fall, she was physically active. However, at the time of the assessment, she was unable to care for or provide for herself. She stated, "Everything was all right when I could walk. Now I'm no use to anyone. All I want to do is die." She stated that she "loved reading" but could no longer do this because of visual problems. She was unable to listen to tapes because of auditory problems. She complained of increasing physical pain. She also complained that her family was deceased or unavailable. Recently, she stopped eating. What action should her physician, the staff at the nursing home, and her family take?

Problems in placement do not always occur. The shrinking woman realized the need for help and voluntarily entered a residential care facility. In cases of physical and mental impairment, the need for care is evident. Such is the situation with Rita.

CASE #30: RITA

Rita was 94 years old when admitted to a nursing home. Prior to that time, she had lived with her family. Most of the problems discussed in Chapter 22 occurred during her stay with the family as her abilities—physical, functional, and cognitive—diminished. Medical problems included cardiovascular disease, cystitis, and "organic brain syndrome." Recently, she had become delusional with paranoid ideations. On one occasion, she threatened to kill a family member with a knife. Neuroleptic medication did not calm her.

Ability to reason and make logical judgments had deteriorated over the years, as had expressive and receptive skills. She was incontinent and unable to care for herself. The diagnosis was late-stage Alzheimer's. The need for intensive care was obvious. Still, the family had a great deal of guilt and pain in placing her in a nursing home.

Bob resisted placement; and there were some questions whether he should have been admitted to a nursing home, as in the case of Mick the Bullet in Chapter 9.

CASE #31: BOB

Prior to admission to a nursing home, Bob (85 years old) lived with his wife. The wife reported that he had become disoriented, confused, irritable, and abusive. While he was physically able to ambulate, he tended to sit in front of the television or stay in bed, making demands of his wife. The wife added that he had a tendency to become easily frustrated. He had few interests and few friends. He refused to allow his wife, who was 83, to obtain outside help. He complained when the wife left the house and refused to allow her to have company. The wife contacted a nursing facility and requested that an evaluation be made, with the hope that her husband would be admitted to the facility. (An evaluation in a case like this should include an assessment of physical, functional, mental, and emotional needs and abilities. Because the individual resists placement, issues of rights, competence, and need arise.) Bob was not suffering from Alzheimer's disease; however, the issue of competence and ability to continue to manage his own affairs had to be addressed.

There are many types of competence under the law, including competence in making contracts and consenting to medical treatment. Competence to manage property and one's financial matters is often an ability that must be assessed. In respect to medical treatment, the individual must be able to understand, among other factors, the consequence of refusing treatment. Psychological assessments are used in court as the basis for determining whether a person can make rational judgments, reason, abstract, test reality, and problem solve.

Power of attorney is a contract or agreement that allows another person to act in one's behalf. General power of attorney covers all areas, whereas specific power of attorney limits the action to specific acts, such as managing financial affairs. The power of attorney may also be limited to a specific time period. Power of attorney can be terminated at any time by the grantor. However, durable power of attorney may be granted, where the power becomes irrevocable in the case of incapacity, either physical or mental.

Because family members must make decisions regarding care and treatment in the case of an individual with Alzheimer's disease, durable power of attorney for health care is often suggested. Bob's wife, following consultation with her attorney, decided to seek durable power of attorney regarding her husband's medical and health care. However, power of attorney requires the consent of the grantor. Bob resisted giving his consent. The wife then applied for guardianship. Guardianship allows for the guardian to act on behalf of an individual who is incapable of managing his or her own affairs because of physical or mental incapacity. It is not uncommon for family members to seek guardianship during the early stage of dementia in the case of another family member. One reason for an early assessment and diagnosis is to provide the family (and, if necessary, the courts) with specific information and data in regard to competency.

Decisions regarding property management and disposition at death should be discussed with experts in the field of law and banking when an individual is diagnosed as suffering from Alzheimer's. Financial planning is important to provide the best of care, with consideration of future costs and projected life span. The needs of the spouse must be taken into account in situations where one marital partner is suffering from dementia.

An individual's rights are protected by law. Patients' rights must be posted in nursing homes as well as hospitals. Ombudsman services or some other form of representation in situations of complaint by either the patient or family must also be available. An ombudsman is one who speaks on behalf of another. The ombudsman must be available on a regular basis. The goal of the ombudsman is to resolve resident complaints, inform residents of rights, provide information on resident need and concerns of the community, and act as an advocate on behalf of residents for changes in laws and policies to improve long term care services.

Ombudsman services may be used by residents, staff and administrators, the community at large, and other interested individuals, including family members. Complaints can also be directed to state and local agencies that accredit, supervise, monitor, and inspect healthcare facilities or providers. State offices on the aging can provide information on ombudsman services, respite resources, and referral services.

Under recent law, nursing homes must protect the following resident rights:

Rights to self-determination

Personal and privacy rights

Rights regarding abuse and restraints

Rights to information

Rights to visits

Transfer and discharge rights

Protection of personal funds

Protection against Medicaid discrimination

Specifics about these rights can be obtained from the nursing home. Nursing homes are also required to provide for its residents "to promote maintenance or enhancement of quality of life" and "to provide services and activities to attain or maintain the highest practical physical, mental, psychosocial well-being of each resident."

Agencies which are involved and concerned about the care and welfare of the elderly include the following:

State Office on Aging
National Institution on Aging
National Institute on Mental Health
Alzheimer's Association
American Association of Retired Persons
American Geriatric Association
American Health-Care Association
American Association of Homes for the Aging
American Medical Association
American Psychological Association
American Society on Aging
Gray Panthers
National Association of Social Workers
National Citizens Coalition for Nursing Home Reform
National Council on Aging

PART IV

CONCURRENT EMOTIONAL AND MENTAL DISORDERS COMMON IN THE ELDERLY

CHAPTER 27

Paranoid Disorders

As discussed in Chapter 7, it is estimated that 18 percent of the individuals who have been diagnosed as suffering from Alzheimer's disease actually suffer from other emotional disorders that present as dementia. This book has emphasized the importance of an accurate diagnosis in order to diagnose, treat, and manage not only Alzheimer's patients but also those with reversible forms of dementia.

Part IV approaches the subject of treatment and management from a different perspective. Studies indicate that patients with dementia may indeed have concurrent or concurring emotional problems and mental disorders that complicate management. It has been suggested that elderly individuals tend to suffer from paranoid disorders, depression, and anxiety disorders at least as commonly as the general population and possibly more often. Personality traits and disorders also tend to become more entrenched with aging and may become more obvious with those suffering from Alzheimer's.

Because these disorders complicate treatment and management, Part IV has been written to improve recognition of the symptoms of paranoia, anxiety disorders, depression, and personality disorders and traits and explore issues related to the elderly. The following discussion is based on criteria from *DSM-IV*.

Paranoia appears to be fairly common in the elderly. One study of ninety-nine patients ages 60 years and older who had been admitted to psychiatric hospitals indicated that 10 percent displayed significant features and symptoms of paranoia. This author's experience supports this statistic based on reports by family and staff in nursing homes.

Commonalities among elderly people who suffer from paranoia include low marriage rates, few surviving relatives, personality traits of suspiciousness and mistrust in early years, and hearing loss. Studies suggest that sensory loss and social isolation or withdrawal tend to contribute to the risk of paranoia. In the case of withdrawal, the question must be asked whether the individual has become isolative because of paranoid thoughts and ideations or whether the isolation has led to mistrust. In the case of hearing loss and loss of other sensory abilities, it is easy to recognize that interpersonal relationships become more difficult and that there develops the risk of misunderstanding and confusion. The individual who cannot see may well develop suspicions that items have been stolen when, in fact, they have been lost or misplaced.

Individuals who have been considered "loners" tend to become more isolative with age. As is discussed in greater depth in Chapter 30, these disorders tend to become more severe and debilitative with age. An individual who has been positive and outgoing throughout life tends to have a positive outlook throughout the aging process. The exception to this tends to be in cases of severe physical illness and in cases of personality change due to organicity. Individuals with Alzheimer's may go through radical personality change during the early and middle stages of the dementia. It has been estimated that 20 percent of the individuals with Alzheimer's dementia suffer from paranoid symptoms.

DSM-IV distinguishes between delusional disorder and paranoid personality disorder. A delusional disorder requires that the individual experience nonbizarre delusions that have existed for at least one month. Examples of these delusions include the belief that an individual is being poisoned; that others are stealing from the individual; that one is being deceived by a spouse or family member; or that one is being followed, spied on, or persecuted. Elderly patients often focus on one particular family member, a staff person in a nursing home, or a neighbor or acquaintance. Issues with the elderly include fear of loss of property, fears of being taken advantage of financially, and fears of personal safety. Usually, these delusions are specific and focal rather than global. These fears and suspicions are commonly related to feelings of loss or lack of power and control as well as dependence on others and fears that basic needs will not be taken care of and met.

DSM-IV criteria for delusional disorder rule out bizarre delusions as are common with schizophrenia. An individual who is suffering from delusional disorder is not necessarily cognitively impaired in other ways. However, when this disorder is coexisting with a form of dementia, there is cognitive impairment. These impairments, such as confusion, problems with abstract thinking and reasoning, and disorientation, are due to organic factors and the dementia. There are various types of delusional disorder:

1. Erotomanic-type delusions, where the delusional individual imagines a love relationship with someone usually of a higher status. It is not uncommon for an individual in an institutional facility to become unrealistically attached to a staff member with the imaging that this attachment is sexual or romantic. Individuals suffering from Alzheimer's do, on occasion, become sexually inappropriate. However, this is more likely because of confusion and impulse control problems than because of delusions.

2. Grandiose-type delusions are those of inflated worth, power, ability, or relationship to a deity or powerful person. Individuals tend to lose their sense of identity and self-worth as the aging process continues. Loss of physical and mental ability, loss of role and importance in the family and community, loss of purpose in life, and loss of mobility are all threats and, in many cases, reality as we age. There is a difference between psychological defense mechanisms where the individual behaves in grandiose, narcissistic, or egocentric ways to compensate for loss and the delusional patient. Distinguishing between delusion-based behavior and nondelusional behavior is important in treatment and management. Delusions are often treated with neuroleptic medication. Helping the nondelusional but demanding family member or patient feel significant, safe, and loved may improve behavior. The individual with dementia also needs love, attention, and feelings of security. As Alzheimer's progresses and cognitive abilities decrease, providing assurance may be more difficult. As has been discussed, verbal reasoning is no longer effective. Providing structure, continuity, and consistency for the individual's physical well being and hygiene become primary.

3. Individuals in early- and late-stage Alzheimer's tend to become very dependent on the spouse or primary caretaker. While jealous delusions are another type of delusional disorder, there may be some question whether the individual suffering from dependency actually suspects infidelity or is merely overly dependent. In situations of jealous delusions, reasoning does not help. Distraction is a good technique to be used by the accused party rather than trying to convince the delusional person of one's fidelity. Overly dependent individuals suffering from Alzheimer's disease will demand constant assurance that their needs will be met. Keeping the environment calm and stable will help ease fears about being abandoned.

4. Persecutory delusions are another form of delusion disorder. Individuals with Alzheimer's tend to be suspicious and paranoid because of confusion, anxiety, and disorientation. Just as patients with Alzheimer's may become attached to a particular staff or family member, those with the disease may have persecutory delusions about one person with whom they have contact. Individuals suffering from persecutory-type delusions may become violent.

5. The central theme of somatic delusions relates to concern about body functions and sensations. Somatic concerns are common with the elderly but often do not meet the criteria to be classified as a delusional disorder.

In the case of delusional disorder, functioning may be relatively unimpaired to severely impaired. Delusional disorders and other forms of psychopathology tend to have a greater dibilitative impact on those individuals with limited support systems and psychological resources. Because of this, the elderly tend to become more dysfunctional and impaired when suffering from such disorders as depression, paranoia, and anxiety. Pre-existing mental disorders tend to become more severe with aging. While it has been suggested that emotional problems and pathology can contribute to physical and medical disorders, it is also likely that being physically ill can result in emotional problems.

Individuals who suffer from Alzheimer's disease (in the opinion of this author, based on extensive clinical experience) tend to be anxious; depressed; and, in some cases, paranoid, especially in the early stage of Alzheimer's. The possibility that these disorders coexist with dementia must be recognized and the symptoms treated.

DSM-IV reports that delusional disorders occur in about 3 percent of the population and that age of onset is usually middle age or late middle age. Late-onset dementia of the Alzheimer's type is classified as occurring after age 65, which suggests that delusions may occur before the onset of dementia. Persecutory delusions are the most common type. The delusional process may be episodic or chronic, and there may be remission. As discussed earlier, with the onset of dementia, the delusions tend to be less specific and less focal.

DSM-IV includes paranoid personality disorder as one of eleven personality disorders. The other personality disorders and issues related to aging, the elderly, and dementia are discussed in Chapter 30.

Paranoid personality disorder is defined as a distrust and suspiciousness of others that is pervasive. The motives of others are interpreted as being malevolent. Symptoms include suspicions of being exploited, preoccupation with doubts of loyalty of friends, reluctance to confide in others because of fear of being treated maliciously, looking for hidden demeaning or harmful meanings in events or remarks, holding of grudges, beliefs that others are attacking one's reputation, and suspicions about fidelity of a significant other or spouse.

Paranoid personality disorder differs from delusional disorder in that there are no delusions or psychotic features. Sometimes, paranoid personality disorder traits develop related to a medical condition; in association with abuse of substances such as alcohol, marijuana, or cocaine; or as the result of physical disabilities.

Paranoid personality disorder is reported among 0.5 to 2.5 percent of the general population. It is probable that a greater percentage of the elderly suffer from paranoid personality disorder traits than this statistic. Aging tends to bring illness; and with physical illness, decompensation and regression are likely. The symptoms of paranoid personality disorder often appear in childhood or adolescence. These symptoms include solitariness, poor peer relationships, anxiety about social involvement, hypersensitivity, and egocentric fantasies. With the aging process, symptoms and behaviors tend to become more entrenched. During early-stage Alzheimer's, they further impair the individual's functioning and create management and interpersonal problems. Individuals with paranoid personality disorder traits have problems with close relationships. Recurrent complaints, argumentativeness, and hostility alienates these individuals from others. Rigidity, the need to be in control of situations and people, and a critical nature are related and associated features. Because of this, one's needs are often not met, with an increase in negative behavior and attitude. Related concurring personality disorders are schizotypal, schizoid, narcissistic, avoidant, and borderline (see Chapter 30).

The following case study is about a woman with paranoid delusional disorder. A neuropsychological assessment was ordered to rule out dementia. The subject was not suffering from dementia. However, imagine the compounding of problems had she been in early-stage Alzheimer's.

CASE #32: DELORES

The subject was an 83-year-old white woman who was living in her own one-bedroom apartment in a retirement setting. The director of social services reported that he had concerns about the individual's anxiety and functional ability. Staff members stated that the subject tended to decompensate easily and was preoccupied with the ideation that a maintenance worker at the facility was harassing her. She stated that the staff worker, who was a male, followed her to the dining room. She continued, "Once he's sure I'm in the dining room, he goes to my room and moves things around." She continued, "One day, he took talcum powder and sprinkled it on the back of my chair. Then he took the container and put it on a shelf in the living room instead of back in the bathroom. Another time, he came into my apartment and clipped all of the berries and flowers off a wreath I had hanging on my door." She also complained that he had taken some of her belongings.

During an interview with the daughter, she stated that the mother had been somewhat avoidant and isolative and that paranoid delusions began about four years ago. The mother had lived in the retirement facility for about seven years, so it was unlikely that a recent move or loss had resulted in exacerbated and more severe symptoms. Because the onset of the more extreme paranoia had been gradual, it could not be ruled out that this was related to organicity. Organic brain damage from a CVA or TIA to the frontal lobes can result in personality change. However, this change is usually acute. In the middle stage of Alzheimer's disease, personality change occurs more gradually.

However, a review of the subject's medical records ruled out vascular dementia. During the assessment, it was determined that the subject was oriented and able to function independently. She was neatly and attractively dressed. Her apartment was clean and organized. While she did display some signs of anxiety, rapport was established; and she was able to relate appropriately. At times, she displayed a good sense of humor.

She was able to recall data and information from her childhood and knew dates and names. She became mildly confused when asked about details; however, this appeared to be related to embarrassment and a desire to perform well. She tended to be a perfectionist. When given time and encouraged, performance improved.

Expressive and receptive language abilities were intact. She did well on the cognitive and neuropsychological tests. However, the delusional ideations were obvious with problems in reality testing. She was convinced that the events described had taken place. When asked to further elaborate, she added more details.

While it appears that this individual has been avoidant, isolative, and suspicious much of her life, the symptoms suggested that her paranoia had become delusional rather than being trait related. Suggestions to the staff for management included encouragement to participate in social and physical activity events to distract her from her preoccupations and delusions. At the time of the assessment, she spent all of the time dwelling on her concerns. Family involvement was also suggested. Staff members were advised to be patient, available, and nonconfrontive. Distraction rather than argument and confrontation is best when dealing with an individual with delusions. Neuroleptic medication might be considered by her physician, with side effects and response monitored.

CHAPTER 28

Anxiety Disorders

Many elderly people suffer from anxiety. In the majority of cases, the symptoms are not severe or extreme enough to result in the classification by *DSM-IV* as an anxiety disorder. However, anxiety can and often does exist where the individual's ability to function is impaired. This chapter discusses the symptoms of anxiety disorders and addresses issues related to management and treatment of subclinical symptoms. Individuals with dementia, in particular, are prone to anxiety symptoms, in large part, because of problems with orientation and confusion. Agitation and tension result from such things as being unsure of what is taking place in one's environment; not remembering names, places, and people; being unable to carry out sequential tasks that were easy to perform in the past; and having to depend on others for basic needs. Individuals who suffer from physical problems and disabilities also tend to develop anxiety symptoms, as do individuals who have suffered losses such as moving from an independent living situation to a nursing home, being unable to drive a car, and being separated from one's community.

Change tends to result in dysphoria and concerns about the future and one's well-being. Even without the loss of cognitive abilities that takes place with Alzheimer's, the elderly tend to be at risk for anxiety. It is important to identify anxiety, not only the type but also the severity and the impact on the individual's functional condition when treating the elderly patient. Treatment of anxiety disorders in the elderly is discussed in Chapters 17 and 18 and includes consideration of psychotropic medication and psychotherapy. Additional information has been provided on management techniques. This chapter focuses on diagnostic criteria, prevalence, course of the disorder, and differential diagnosis of anxiety disorders in the adult population. *DSM-IV* also discusses anxiety disorders of childhood and adolescence, which are not addressed in this book.

The most prevalent mental disorder suffered by adults is anxiety disorder. Panic disorder is the most common subtype. Studies indicate that the prevalence of panic disorder is between 1.5 and 3.5 percent of the population. This translates to 4 to 8 million Americans suffering from this form of anxiety disorder.

According to *DSM-IV*, a panic attack is defined as "a discrete period of intense fear or discomfort." During this period, certain symptoms develop. These can include heart palpitations, sweating, shaking, shortness of breath, chest pain, a sensation of choking, nausea, dizziness, feelings of unreality, fear of loss of control, fear of dying, numbness of extremities, and chills or hot flashes. Panic disorder is classified either with agoraphobia, which results in anxiety about being in places where escape might be difficult or embarrassing or in which needed help might not be available, or without agoraphobia, in which these fears are not present. *DSM-IV* also lists the disorder agoraphobia without a history of panic attacks. In order for attacks to be classified as panic disorder, the attacks must be recurrent and unexpected and at least one of the panic attacks followed by one month or more of either persistent concern about having additional attacks, worry about the implications or consequences of an attack, or a significant change in behavior as the result of the attacks.

There are no statistics on the prevalence of panic disorder among the elderly, in general, and among those suffering from dementia of the Alzheimer's type, specifically. However, it is speculated that of the percentage of individuals in the general population suffering from panic attacks (1.5% to 3.5%), a high percentage suffer from panic disorder.

Too often, anxiety among the elderly is not properly diagnosed and treated. The symptoms may be considered to be either insignificant or situational when, indeed, the elderly parent or patient is suffering from a distinct and specific type of mental disorder that can and should be treated. Often, this disorder is preexisting yet becomes more severe and debilitating with change, loss, or insecurity.

It is not uncommon for family members, significant others, and caretakers to encourage the individual suffering from panic disorder to become more socially involved. Engagement theory, which is discussed in Chapters 20 and 21, suggests the benefits of social involvement, and many of the recommendations made in case studies in this book focus on the need to stay socially involved and active. However, this is not always beneficial. In the case of individuals suffering from panic disorder, avoidant personality disorder, or dementia, social involvement may lead to decompensation and exacerbation of pathology. This emphasizes the need for a complete and accurate evaluation and assessment of an individual's mental and emotional state and situation.

Just as major depression presents symptoms similar to dementia, anxiety disorders can result in disorientation, confusion, problems with attention and concentration, and thought-processing problems. Being aware of the symptoms of panic disorder will allow the diagnostician, mental health professional, and other caretakers to respond in therapeutic and helpful ways.

The frequency and severity of panic attacks tend to vary from individual to individual. Some individuals experience partial remission, while others have panic attacks that occur regularly for long periods of time. Some individuals experience limited-symptom attacks, while others experience full panic attacks. Many individuals become withdrawn because of fear of embarrassment or fear of the consequences of an attack. During the early stages of Alzheimer's, fear of embarrassment is also common. However, the condition experienced by the individual is probably generalized anxiety rather than panic per se. As Alzheimer's progresses, anxiety becomes agitation. Individuals in middle- to late-stage Alzheimer's do not have the analytical ability to focus on particulars. They tend to be generally confused and disoriented rather than anxious about a particular situation, person, or object.

Individuals suffering from panic disorder are excessively apprehensive or concerned about specifics, such as the outcome of a particular event or situation, or the health and well-being of a loved one. Catastrophic outcomes are anticipated. Another associated feature of panic disorder is demoralization, where the individual feels ashamed or discouraged. Anxiety often leads to depression. It is estimated that from 50 to 65 percent of the individuals with panic disorder suffer from major depression.

Age of onset for panic disorder is most commonly between late adolescence and the mid-30s. The course tends to vary throughout one's lifetime yet is typically chronic. Thus, it would appear that a family history and inquiry into past mental problems would be primary when treating an elderly individual and as a part of need, care, and management planning in a residential setting. Individuals who are suffering from Alzheimer's disease with a past history of anxiety disorder may have special needs. During the early stages of Alzheimer's these patients tend to become more easily upset and agitated. Providing a calm, stable, low-stimulation environment and setting tends to diminish agitation and anxiety. (See discussion on management techniques in Chapters 20 and 21.)

Other subtypes of anxiety disorder include specific phobia disorder, social phobia, obsessive–compulsive disorder, posttraumatic stress and acute stress disorder, generalized anxiety disorder, anxiety disorder due to general medical condition, and substance-induced anxiety disorder.

Generalized anxiety is defined as excessive anxiety and worry or apprehensive expectation. The anxiety must occur for at least six months, with the anxiety being present more days than not. An associated feature is difficulty in controlling the worry. Specific symptoms include restlessness, fatigue, problems with concentration, irritability, muscle tension, and sleep disturbance. In order to be classified as generalized anxiety, there must be significant distress or impairment in major life areas. In cases of generalized anxiety disorder, the intensity, duration, and frequency of the anxiety is out of proportion to normal worry or concern. Because of preoccupation with concerns, the individual has problems completing everyday tasks. Associated features include somatic symptoms and exaggerated startle response. The problems with attention, functional ability, concentration, and task completion are similar to problems observed in early-stage Alzheimer's, again emphasizing the importance of an accurate diagnosis based on a comprehensive evaluation and assessment. Generalized anxiety disorder may coexist with dementia.

It is estimated that at any one time, approximately 35 percent of the population has experienced generalized anxiety. A closely related form of psychopathology is adjustment disorder with anxiety. While many of the symptoms are similar to generalized anxiety, there exists an identified stressor or stressors within three months of the onset of adjustment disorder with anxiety. DSM-IV also identifies adjustment disorder with depressed mood, with mixed anxiety and depressed mood, with disturbance of conduct, and with mixed disturbance of emotions and conduct.

Anxiety, which can present symptoms similar to dementia, appears to be relatively common among elderly who have experienced loss, changes, and disappointment. Having to move from the family home, the death of a spouse, or a physical disability are examples of stressors that can cause an adjustment disorder.

Anxiety due to a general medical condition is also fairly common among the elderly. The essential feature of this disorder is that the anxiety is considered to be due to the direct physiological effects of a general medical condition. In order for this to be a diagnosis, there must be evidence from history, physical examination, or laboratory testing. Endocrine, cardiovascular, respiratory, metabolic, and neurological conditions can all be causal factors.

Another subtype of anxiety is social phobia, where the individual has a persistent fear of social situations. This is similar to panic disorder, only with a specific fear of social events. This disorder obviously causes avoidant personality behaviors. An associated feature is performance phobia, sometimes known as "stage fright," in which the individual fears exposure to unfamiliar people or possible scrutiny by others in performance situations. The nursing home resident who refuses to eat in the public dining room may be suffering from social phobia, although many individuals in early stages of Alzheimer's are aware of their cognitive and functional problems and avoid social situations and events. Estimates of prevalence of social phobia range from 3 to 13 percent of the population, depending on the criteria and particular study. Age of onset is typically the mid-teens. Thus, elderly patients who suffer from this anxiety disorder have probably been lifetime sufferers. Mere encouragement to socialize will probably not meet with much success. As was suggested in cases of panic disorder, caretakers must be practical in realizing that behavioral and attitudinal changes will not be significant in later years. Accommodations should be made with an emphasis on respecting the rights and dignity of the individual.

Individuals with dementia may exhibit obsessive–compulsive symptoms. There may also be signs of psychosis. Obsessive–compulsive disorder differs from obsessive–compulsive behaviors related to dementia in that there is no gross thought disorder and that the individual realizes that the obsessive thoughts or compulsive impulses are a product of his or her own mind. The individual suffering from the disorder attempts to suppress or ignore the impulses and thoughts. Last, their thoughts and impulses cause marked distress. Obsessive–compulsive symptoms related to stress may be observed in nursing homes. Again, it is important to determine if such behavior is related to psychosis, dementia, or stress.

Specific phobia includes fear or avoidance of animals or insects; fear of natural environment objects or situations such as storms, heights, or water; fear of blood, injection, or physical injury; and fear of situations involving tunnels, bridges, elevators, flying, enclosed spaces, or driving. An anxiety response takes place on exposure to phobic stimuli. In the case of a specific phobia, the sufferer experiences intense anxiety or distress and realizes that the fear is excessive. Although phobic behavior or response may be moderately common in the general public, reaction is seldom sufficient to meet the criteria of intense anxiety or distress.

SUMMARY

This chapter has focused on various subtypes of anxiety disorder. It is suggested that the elderly may suffer from the symptoms of anxiety more often than the general population because of losses; fears about the future; loneliness; lack of goal, direction, and a meaning in life; or physical illness or disability.

Anxiety may be severe and result in cognitive and functional impairment similar to dementia. Anxiety may be secondary to other forms of mental illness or primary. It may result from psychosocial stressors or be chronic. It may also be pre-existing or concurrent with dementia. In any case, anxiety disorder symptoms should be noted and a diagnosis ordered to ascertain the extent, severity, and the cause and make recommendations for treatment. Available treatment techniques include pharmacological intervention, psychotherapy, and behavior-modification techniques.

CHAPTER 29

Major Depressive Disorders

This chapter discusses major depression and the aging population. Studies indicate that the lifetime risk for major depression in the general population varies from 10 to 25 percent in women to 5 to 12 percent in men. However, there appears to be a higher frequency rate among the elderly. Major depression in the elderly population is often not diagnosed because of the misconception that depressive disorders are a natural phenomenon in the aging process and related to dementia.

This, in fact, is not true. Often, clinical depression is primary, although the symptoms can be similar to those observed in dementia. Much has been written in this book about depression and the need for an accurate diagnosis. Treatment of depression may eliminate problems with memory, concentration, attention, judgment, and orientation. When pre-existing or coexisting depression is not diagnosed and treated, functional and cognitive impairment due to dementia tend to increase and become more severe.

DSM-IV lists a number of symptoms that may be present during a two-week cycle and that represent a change from previous functioning as the criteria for a major depressive episode. These include the following:

1. A depressed mood most of the day, nearly every day
2. Significant decrease in interest or pleasure in activities
3. Significant weight gain or loss or decrease or increase in appetite
4. Insomnia or hypersomnia
5. Psychomotor agitation or retardation
6. Energy loss or fatigue
7. Feelings of worthlessness or inappropriate guilt

8. Problems with thinking and concentration or indecisiveness
9. Recurrent thoughts of death or suicide or a suicide attempt or plan

At least five of these symptoms must exist nearly every day for a two-week period to meet the diagnosis of major depression. These symptoms must cause significant stress or functional impairment. Sadness and normal grieving are not considered to be major depression.

Often, individuals suffering from major depression deny the symptoms, discount or minimize their distress, or try to rationalize or explain away their behavior. The elderly, who often have problems with disclosure or admitting emotional symptoms, present a real challenge to the diagnostician. An accurate diagnosis of depression may also be difficult because of existing general medical conditions, such as cancer, stroke, diabetes, or myocardial infarction, which may have similar features. Also, symptoms of dementia are similar to symptoms of depression. Just as a depressed patient may be diagnosed as suffering from dementia, a patient with dementia may be diagnosed as suffering from major depression. The preceding chapters emphasize the need for an accurate diagnosis as well as discuss diagnostic techniques and methods.

Associated features of major depression include tearfulness, irritability, obsessive thinking, anxiety, excessive worry over health, and psychosomatic pain. Headaches, backaches, and abdominal pain are common. Many of these symptoms are complaints of the elderly but do not necessarily qualify one to be diagnosed as depressed. As of January 1996, no laboratory test or findings have been developed to diagnose major depression. However, laboratory tests are useful to rule out physical and medical conditions that may present major depressive symptoms, just as laboratory tests should be utilized in ruling out medical conditions that present as dementia of the Alzheimer's type.

The importance of an accurate diagnosis related to major depression is emphasized by the high mortality rate associated with the disorder. Up to 15 percent of those suffering from major depression commit suicide. The depressed elderly patient is at real risk. A history of psychosis, chronic depression, substance abuse, and previous inpatient treatment are all increased risk factors, as are such stressors as loss of a spouse, severe medical problems, and loss of significant support systems. Severely depressed individuals on antidepressant medication should be monitored because of the risk of overdosing. Elderly patients suffering from confusion or dementia should also be monitored, with medications supervised. The severely depressed individual is also at risk for sedative and tranquilizer overdose.

The severity of major depression varies from mild to severe. Psychotic symptoms may be observed. Major depression may be in partial remission or full remission. Other specifics of the depression noted in *DSM-IV* include chronicity with catatonic, melancholic, or atypical features; with postpartum onset; with or without interepisode recovery; and with a seasonal pattern.

The degree of dysfunction and impairment experienced by the patient depends on, among other factors, the severity of the depression, the resources of the individual, one's support system, and treatment. Elderly individuals frequently suffer a number of stressors and experience a number of changes and losses at the same time. Of the ten most stressful lifetime events or situations, the elderly are overexposed to four. These are the death of a spouse (the most extreme stressful event [#1]), the death of a close family member (#5), personal injury or illness (#6), and retirement (#10). Other top-ten stressors include divorce, marital separation, incarceration, marriage, being fired from a job, and marital reconciliation.

The elderly are also at risk for severe depression because of limited resources. These include financial, physical, mental, and emotional resources. Physical illness and disability may result in depression not only because of loss of mobility, pain, and inconvenience but also because resources and the ability to deal with daily life situations are depleted. With dementia come problems in analyzing situations, in executive functioning, and in relating to others. As discussed previously, individuals in early-stage Alzheimer's tend to be depressed; and this depression is commonly secondary. However, major depression may be primary and coexisting. Individuals also are more at risk for depression as the aging process takes place, in situations where support systems are not available. Moving an individual from a familiar neighborhood or community to a nursing home may result in depression. Abandonment of the elderly by family can also lead to depression. Recently, abuse of the elderly by family caretakers has received attention in the media, although it has most likely existed for a long time.

Family stress develops when adults must assume responsibility for an aging parent, especially when the adults have children of their own to provide care. Reversal of roles, financial and time demands, and loss of parent issues are all involved. Stress increases in the case of a bedridden elderly parent or one with a disorder such as Alzheimer's, especially when no relief is provided. Statistics reveal that parent abuse tends to increase in the elderly over age 75, with elderly women more likely to be abused than elderly men.

Major depressive disorder can begin at any time in the life span; however, the average age of onset is in the 20s. Thus, many of the elderly patients who suffer from depression are chronic sufferers. However, as discussed earlier, depression in the elderly can be acute or episodes may become more frequent or more severe. More than 50 percent of the individuals who experience one episode of major depression are expected to experience a second episode. Of individuals who have second episodes, 70 percent are at risk of having a third episode. Episodes are likely to follow significant psychosocial stressors, which accounts for the prevalence of major depression in the elderly following loss or change. There appears to be a genetic predisposition for major depression disorder with the disorder from 1.5 to 3 times more common among first-degree biological relatives than among the general population.

Another mental disorder closely resembling major depression is dysthymic disorder. The distinguishing symptom of this disorder is a chronically depressed mood that occurs daily or most of the days over a two-year period. Symptoms include at least two of the following in order to be classified as dysthymic disorder:

1. Poor appetite or overeating
2. Insomnia or hypersomnia
3. Low energy or fatigue
4. Low self-esteem
5. Problems with concentration or indecisiveness
6. Feelings of hopelessness

These symptoms must cause significant distress or functional impairment.

Often, individuals suffering from dysthymic disorder portray themselves as chronically depressed and see change as hopeless. Associated features may include feelings of inadequacy and guilt, a general loss of interest in life, social withdrawal, irritability, and anger. Vegetative symptoms are less common for persons suffering from dysthymic disorder than major depression disorder. About 6 percent of the general population will suffer from dysthymic disorder at one time or another in their life. There appears to be a familial pattern for dysthymic disorder.

DSM-IV lists a number of other mood disorders, including bipolar disorder. The significant feature of bipolar disorder is that the individual suffering from the disorder has experienced one or more manic or hypomanic episodes. More information can be obtained about this particular form of mood disorder from DSM-IV. The discussion in this book is limited to depressive and dysthymic disorders because these disorders are more prevalent in the general population and, in the experience of this author, more common among the elderly.

The following case studies are included to illustrate the difference between dementia and depression. The subject in the first case study is suffering from dementia but is not clinically depressed.

CASE #33: DORA

Dora was 89 years old when tested for dementia and related emotional problems. She had been living in a nursing home for about two years. An assessment was requested because of staff concern about management problems and the resident's high state of agitation. The individual tended to wander and became very upset after visits with family and relatives. She also had made allegations that a male staff member was being sexually inappropriate with her (see Chapter 27 on delusional paranoid disorders).

At the time of the neuropsychological assessment, the patient was taking a neuroleptic medication and an antidepressant. There appears to be a tendency to prescribe an antidepressant for elderly nursing home residents even though they often have not been adequately tested for mood disorder. This case illustrates how dementia can and often does exist without concurrent depression. It may be argued that diagnostic work is time consuming and costly and that prescribing antidepressant medication should be done as a matter of course. This argument is indicative of the lack of care often provided elderly patients. All medications have side effects and should be prescribed with caution, especially when treating elderly patients. The particular antidepressant drug prescribed this 89-year-old woman is known to have anticholinergic, sedative, hypotensive, and cardiotoxicity side effects. The patient's medical chart indicated that she was suffering from hypertension and congestive heart failure. The physician's treatment appears to be a good example of negative iatrogenic treatment.

The subject was frail and wore glasses and hearing aids. She was alert but poorly oriented. Her level of anxiety was high. She was able to understand some of the directions and questions yet had problems with word finding, completing tasks, and analytical reasoning. Memory impairment was moderate to severe. As the procedure continued, she became more confused and the extent of her cognitive disabilities became more apparent. The subject had problems with expressive language, suggesting that there may have been some vascular damage. Family members reported, however, that her deterioration had been progressive over a period of about three years.

However, the individual was not depressed. She reported that "everything was fine." Although it was impossible to use all of the psychological instruments and techniques which might have been desirable to test mood, it was determined that the primary diagnosis was dementia. The neuroleptic medication appeared to be appropriate on a prn basis to control agitation and anxiety. The medication chosen was low on anticholinergic side effects and the dosage appropriate.

Recommendations included continued family involvement but on a limited basis, with only one or two members present at one time to guard against overstimulation. The subject appeared to be relatively happy and content in that her family continued to supply love and attention even when the patient was somewhat confused and not always sure of names and relationship. At times, she thought her son was her husband; but she was perfectly happy to sit and hold his hand and was appropriate when he stated that he had to leave. Students, medical and mental health professionals, and others involved in geriatric medicine and mental health would benefit from spending time in a dementia unit at a health-care facility to observe and learn how patients with dementia relate and communicate. Too often, it is assumed that Alzheimer's patients do not respond to love, attention, tactile stimulation, hugging, music, and special care.

Other recommendations included keeping the environment stable and calm, using distraction rather than confrontation, and encouraging participation in simple activities.

CASE #34: ELAINE

The subject was a 65-year-old woman with a number of medical problems, resulting in severe disability. Her medical chart stated that she suffers from "cervical myelopathy, osteoarthritis, spinal cord disease NOS, depression, anxiety, and dementia." She was admitted to a nursing home because her disabilities made independent living and self-care impossible. About six weeks prior to the neuropsychological assessment, the subject's father had died. The father also resided in the same nursing home. Staff members reported that the 65-year-old woman had become psychotic, delusional, and severely depressed. Among other symptoms, they reported those which are common with dementia. The subject reportedly could not concentrate or attend. She was agitated and disoriented as well as grossly confused. She spoke of suicide and expressed feelings of hopelessness, helplessness, and despair. The staff reported that she refused to eat and did not sleep well. She was irritable, restless, and fearful.

When tested, she was in a wheelchair and had limited use of her body. She was able to speak and move her arms and hands slightly, however. Initially, she was resistant to testing. Once rapport was established, she became cooperative. It was obvious that whoever had made the diagnosis of "dementia" was in error. The subject's grief, depression, and anxiety had resulted in problems; however, there were no signs of organicity. She was able to express herself well when given time and encouraged to talk about her past experiences and her feelings. She expressed the belief during the clinical interview that her father had died with Alzheimer's and the fear that she, too, would develop the disorder. This fear exacerbated and contributed to her anxiety and depression. Just as the subject in the Prologue of this book (Anna) began believing that, indeed, she was suffering from dementia, Elaine became vigilant and overly preoccupied with the possibility that she, too, would soon be unable to think and function. She reported that she had been informed that she was "having problems thinking" and that staff members were "concerned about her."

Although she did have problems with memory, attention, and concentration and was, at times, confused and disoriented, her problems were not caused by dementia but, more accurately, by depression and anxiety.

CHAPTER 30

Personality Disorders

DSM-IV lists ten specific personality disorders plus one identified as "personality disorder not otherwise specified." This chapter discusses nine of the personality disorders, for Chapter 27 focused on paranoid personality disorder.

A personality disorder is defined in *DSM-IV* as "an enduring pattern of inner experience and behavior that deviates markedly from the expectations of the individual's culture, is pervasive and inflexible, has an onset in adolescence or early adulthood, is stable over time and leads to distress or impairment." A key phrase is "leads to distress or impairment." Personality disorders are discussed at this time because they may become more severe with age. A person with a personality disorder is usually very difficult to deal with and tends to persist in annoying, disturbing, and dysfunctional behaviors. Social, family, and career usually suffer. As the individual ages, stress, poor health, and loss of purpose and direction can lead to greater demands on significant others and irrational and pathological responses. Usually, individuals who suffer from personality disorders do not seek professional help or treatment. When they do, they are often noncompliant, drop out of treatment, and resist change. They tend to be in denial, rationalize their behaviors, and blame others. When personality disorders coexist with dementia, management and treatment tend to be made more difficult. Many of the case histories in this book identify personality disorder as a secondary and complicating diagnosis. Some of the individuals have personality disorder traits, which indicates that, while pathology and impairment exist, they may not be severe enough to result in the diagnosis of "disorder." Personality traits are defined in *DSM-IV* as "enduring patterns of perceiving, relating to and thinking about the environment and oneself that are exhibited in a wide range of social and personal contexts." They may be negative or positive. When they are rigid, inflexible, and maladaptive, they can cause real problems.

The elderly parent with antisocial personality disorder traits will probably not respond well to group living and most certainly will resist professional help, especially an assessment of emotional, cognitive, and social ability and possible impairment. This complicates the situation where the individual may be displaying symptoms of dementia. It takes the cooperation of the family and the patience and expertise of the diagnostician to persuade such an individual about the need and benefit from an evaluation.

The individual suffering from avoidant personality traits is also difficult to diagnose and treat because of fear of scrutiny and social conflict. However, if the individual is suffering from dementia, the tendency to stay isolative and withdrawn becomes more extreme. Narcissistic and histrionic personality disorder traits result in frustration for family members, caretakers, and professional health-care and mental health-care professionals. These are just a few of the examples of how individuals suffering from personality disorders and traits complicate diagnosis and treatment.

The diagnosis of personality disorder focuses on long-term functioning and requires not only observation but also supporting data from significant others. Family members may confuse symptoms of dementia with personality disorder traits; thus, it is important, when dementia is suspected, to assess the individual's cognitive abilities and emotional state using a comprehensive battery (see Chapters 8 to 15). Diagnosis is further complicated by the fact that family members may no longer consider dysfunctional behavior as problematic. Poor hygiene, poorly developed organizational or living skills, social isolation, and other dysfunctional behaviors and responses may be signs of dementia; but these may be overlooked in the context of accepting the individual's behavior or trying to accept their behavior over the years.

In making diagnostic judgments about what is to be considered maladaptive behavior, the individual's cultural, social, and ethnic background must be considered. The same is true in the diagnosis of Alzheimer's disease. Individuals who have not adapted to this culture often display behaviors and attitudes which might be judged as inappropriate, strange, or maladaptive when indeed the behavior is appropriate in another culture, setting, or environment.

Personality disorders and traits tend to be exacerbated by physical illness and stress. Individuals experiencing the first stages of dementia of the Alzheimer's type tend to be aware of disorientation, confusion, memory loss, and functional incapacity or disability. This is obviously stressful. With the withdrawal of support systems; changes in life situation, such as moving into a nursing home; and leaving a familiar situation and setting, dementia also tends to become severe.

Some types of personality disorders, such as antisocial personality and borderline personality disorders, tend to become less severe with age. However, stress can reverse this process. Males tend to experience antisocial personality disorder more frequently than females. Women, on the other hand, are more prone to borderline, narcissistic, histrionic, and dependent personality disorders.

The general criteria for the diagnosis of personality disorder specify four areas of deviation from the norm: (1) cognition and how one perceives and interprets self and the environment; (2) effect or the range, intensity, and appropriate emotional response; (3) interpersonal functioning and one's ability to relate to others in healthy and appropriate ways; and (4) control of impulse. In reviewing these four areas, it becomes evident how deviant personality disorder behaviors, attitudes, and traits resemble many of the symptoms of dementia. Individuals who are disoriented judge the self and the environment in abnormal ways. During early-stage Alzheimer's, emotional instability, lability, and intensity are often out of the norm, with personality change common in middle-stage Alzheimer's. Interpersonal relations are commonly disturbed because of functional and cognitive impairments. Lack of impulse control develops as dementia progresses. A skilled and experienced diagnostician should be able to distinguish dementia from personality disorder; however, a casual observer would have problems, with the personality disorder symptoms tending to mask dementia.

Paranoid personality disorder symptoms have been discussed. Schizoid personality disorder is a pervasive detachment from social relationships and limited emotional range of expression in interpersonal settings. The individual is often described as cold, aloof, and uncaring. This person does not desire or appear to require close personal friends or relationships. They have little interest in sexual activities and seem to be indifferent to praise or criticism. Affect is usually flat, with limited emotional response or expression. Schizoid personality disorder is relatively rare. These individuals may function adequately when allowed to live isolated lives but do poorly in group and social situations, with the possibility of psychotic response when forced to make radical change. It is likely that some individuals in group living situations who act out in angry and sometimes irrational ways are not suffering from psychosis or dementia in a diagnostic sense but are indeed suffering from schizoid personality disorder.

Schizotypal personality disorder is defined as a pattern of social and interpersonal deficits with limited relationships and cognitive and perceptive distortions and eccentric behavior. Symptoms include delusions, odd beliefs and magical thinking, bodily illusions, odd speech, suspicious or paranoid ideation, inappropriate affect, lack of close friends, and excessive social anxiety. Again, some of these symptoms are similar to dementia and or psychosis. Adjustment to group living is difficult for individuals suffering from this disorder also, as it is for individuals with antisocial personality disorder. From 30 to 50 percent of individuals suffering from schizotypal personality disorder suffer from major depression. It has been estimated that about 3 percent of the general population suffer from schizotypal personality disorder. The course of this disorder tends to be stable with the disorder chronic.

From the age of 15, approximately 3 percent of the male population and 1 percent of the female population suffer from antisocial personality disorder, which is described as a pervasive pattern of violation and disregard of the rights of others. Symptoms include refusal to follow social norms and performing acts that constitute breaking the law; continual deceitfulness for purposes of personal gain; impulsivity; irritability and aggressive behavior; disregard for the safety of self and others; work and financial irresponsibility; and lack of remorse for antisocial behaviors and attitudes. Drug abuse and dependence is common with anxiety and major depressive disorder, and pathological gambling and other impulse-control disorders are frequent. While the disorder tends to be chronic, the severity commonly decreases with age. However, individuals with this disorder can be difficult to manage and treat in old age.

Individuals who suffer from borderline personality disorder have unstable interpersonal relations, have problems with self-image, and act from impulse and emotion. Symptoms include fear of abandonment; intense but unhealthy relationships; disturbances of identity; self-damaging impulsivity in such areas as sex, financial matters, and substance abuse; recurrent suicidal or self-mutilating behaviors, thoughts, or gestures; a tendency to overreact emotionally with mood lability; continuing feelings of emptiness; problems controlling anger; and stress-related paranoia.

Individuals with this disorder trait tend to undermine their own success and happiness. Psychotic features are not uncommon. Coexisting disorders frequently include mood disorders, substance abuse, bulimia, posttraumatic stress disorder, and attention deficit disorder. About 2 percent of the population suffer from borderline personality disorder. The more common course of the disorder is chronic instability. Risk of suicide is greatest in early adult years. Some stability occurs with the majority of the individuals with borderline personality disorder in their 30s and 40s. There appears to be a familial pattern in this disorder. Individuals who suffer from this disorder often enter therapy yet present real problems because of broken commitments, resistance, and mood lability. Testing for dementia is usually resisted. Management of individuals with coexisting borderline personality disorder and Alzheimer's is difficult because of instability of mood, a tendency toward passive–aggressive behavior, and outbursts of anger. A tendency for psychotic-like responses and episodes further complicates interpersonal relationships, diagnosis, management, and treatment. As discussed earlier, as Alzheimer's progresses vegetative patterns tend to develop.

The essential feature of histrionic personality disorder is excessive emotional response and attention-seeking behavior. Individuals with this disorder crave attention. Their interactions with others are often shallow and superficial. Sexually inappropriate or provocative behavior is common. Emotional lability is another symptom. Individuals tend to use physical appearance to draw attention to themselves. They exaggerate emotional expression and dramatize themselves. They tend to be easily influenced by others and consider relationships more intimate than usually is the case. Their emotional immaturity and egocentric focus make healthy relationships difficult. They tend to suffer from a variety of other personality disorders, adding to their maladaptive behaviors and attitudes. They tend to crave excitement and have problems completing tasks and living up to commitments. About 2 to 3 percent of the population suffer from this disorder. Associated features include a tendency to focus on physical and medical problems, playing the role of victim, manipulation of others, and alienation from friends because of the constant demand for attention. Histrionic and narcissistic personality disorders have many traits in common.

Narcissistic personality disorder is defined as a pervasive pattern of grandiosity with a need for admiration. Achievement and talent are exaggerated. The individual has fantasies of fame, success, and power and believes that he or she possesses special abilities. These individuals have a sense of entitlement and are exploitive of others. They lack empathy, envy others who are more successful, and tend to be arrogant and aloof. Often, they act with rage and anger when not acknowledged. They reject direction and criticism. About 1 percent of the general population suffer from this disorder.

Individuals with avoidant personality disorder are socially inhibited and experience feelings of inadequency. They are overly sensitive to the criticism of others. They avoid occupations that require social contact, and they are frequently limited in their careers. They resist interpersonal relationships because they fear rejection or being ridiculed or shamed. They believe themselves to be socially inadequate, unappealing physically, and inferior. They resist trying new activities because of fear of failure and shame. Individuals with this disorder tend to become more isolated and withdrawn with aging. Because of this, their support systems and network of those who might be available for company and assistance become smaller. In group living situations, they avoid social contact and interaction. Major depression is common with feelings of loneliness and alienation. Friends are desired; however, their fears interfere with taking the risks involved in interpersonal relationships. Between 0.5 and 1 percent of the population suffer from this disorder.

The significant feature of dependent personality disorder is the excessive need to be taken care of by another, resulting in submissive behavior. The individual with this disorder resists making everyday decisions, allows others to take responsibility for his or her happiness and life, is nonassertive, has problems initiating projects, fears independence, and fears abandonment. Individuals in early-stage Alzheimer's have many of these symptoms because of failing cognitive and functional abilities. It is common for an individual with dementia to depend on one specific family member, although this dependency may be tempered with a demanding attitude and tone. Individuals in early-stage dementia of the Alzheimer's type tend to be angry about their dependence as well as confused about the relationship. In a marital relationship, where responsibilities and decisions were shared, the partner with Alzheimer's may feel a loss of control and trust. Paranoia is common, with accusations of mismanagement and mistreatment based on problems with reality testing and analytical judgment and reasoning. Memory problems can lead to misplaced personal items and belongings, leading to pervasive mistrust and suspiciousness. Thus, the problems of the caretaker increase. Superimposed or preexisting mental disorders make the tasks of caretaking even more difficult.

The last personality disorder listed in *DSM-IV* other than the catch-all diagnostic category personality disorder not otherwise specified is obsessive–compulsive personality disorder, with a pattern of preoccupation with orderliness, perfection, and control. Individuals with this disorder are difficult to interact with because of their rigidity and lack of empathy. About 1 percent of the population suffer from this disorder.

Part IV of this book has been included to provide the reader with very basic information about mental disorders that may coexist with dementia or preexist. The presence of these disorders complicates diagnosis, treatment, and management. In cases of coexistence or preexistence of another disorder, a dual diagnosis should be made and the coexisting disorder treated. This requires skill and experience in areas of pharmacology, health and mental health treatment, and intervention. The following case study is an example of coexisting pathologies.

CASE #35: SARA

The subject is a 67-year-old woman who was admitted to a nursing home following a CVA. She suffered from right-side paralysis yet refused physical and occupational therapy. She also was becoming abusive to the staff and refused to eat. At times, she became physically aggressive, agitated, and hyperverbal.

The patient's family reported that she had a history of alcohol abuse and led the life of a recluse for the last twenty years. At one time, she had been a successful attorney. According to her family, she never married and most of her life lived with her father who was also an attorney. She had few contacts and spent most of her time with her father. With the father's death about twenty years ago, she stopped practicing law and moved into her own apartment. According to her family, she gradually became more distrustful of others and eventually refused visitors and contact with the real world. Concern for the subject's well-being resulted in a cousin obtaining power of attorney. The cousin discovered that the subject was living in unsanitary conditions and made arrangements for her to move to a residential care facility. Prior to the move, the patient suffered a stroke.

The neuropsychological assessment resulted in the diagnosis of vascular dementia. Memory was impaired. The individual had problems with word finding and precision of expression. These impairments appeared to be related to the CVA. However, some expressive language skills had been spared. There were not signs of progressive dementia as would be expected from Alzheimer's. Incremental learning was intact, with the ability to respond to cues and learn new information. She was also alert and oriented. However, abuse of alcohol and personality disorder traits, behaviors, and attitudes resulted in poor cognitive and functional ability. The resulting diagnoses were vascular dementia, major depression (moderate), alcohol dependence, and paranoid and narcissistic personality disorder traits. Management and treatment will be challenging. Recommendations included the use of neuroleptic medication to control anxiety and acting out behaviors, the consideration of using antidepressant medication, psychotherapy to set limits, the development of a management plan, family involvement to relieve the family of feelings of guilt and explore issues of codependency, encouragement in participation in physical therapy, and recognition that alcohol abuse and personality disorder traits exist and probably will not change radically. Setting of limits will be primary. The staff and family should be honest and direct but also supportive.

CONCLUSION

As the American population ages, an increased number of people will suffer from Alzheimer's disease. This book has been written to help students, clinicians, and health-care providers recognize the symptoms of the disease and realize the need for an accurate diagnosis. It is hoped that the book will also result in improved treatment and management of the disorder. While this publication is primarily a textbook, it is intended that there will be some benefit to family members of those suffering from Alzheimer's by improving quality of care and knowledge about this disease.

» «
=====

Bibliography

American Psychiatric Association. *The Diagnostic and Statistical Manual of Mental Disorders*. 4th ed. Washington, D.C.: American Psychiatric Association, 1994.

Battistin, L., and F. Gerstenbrand. *The Aging Brain and the Dementias and Therapy*. New York: Wiley–Liss, 1990.

Bayles, Kathryn A. *The ABC's of Dementia*. Tuscon, Ariz.: Canyonlands, 1993.

Burns, Alstair S. *Clinical Diversity in Late Onset Alzheimer's Disease*. New York: Oxford University Press, 1992.

Cohen, Gene D. *Dementia and Normal Aging*. New York: Cambridge University Press, 1994.

Cummings, J. L., and B. L. Miller, eds. *Alzheimer's Disease: Treatment and Long Term Management*. New York: Dekker Press, 1990.

Cusdorph, H. Richard. *Toxic Metal Syndrome*. Garden City, N.J.: Avery Publications, 1995.

Cutler, Neal R. *Alzheimer's Disease: Optimizing Drug Development Strategies*. New York: Wiley, 1994.

Cutler, Neal R., ed. *Alzheimer's Disease: Clinical Treatment Perspectives*. New York: Wiley, 1995.

Deecke, L., and P. DalBianco, eds. *Age-Associated Neurological Diseases*. New York: Wien, 1991.

Dippel, R. L., and J. T. HuHon, eds. *Caring for the Alzheimer's Patient: A Practical Guide*. Buffalo, N.Y.: Prometheus Books, 1991.

Dowling, James R. *Keeping Busy: Handbook for Persons with Dementia*. Baltimore: Johns Hopkins University Press, 1995.

Edwards, Allen Jack. *When Memory Fails: Helping the Alzheimer's and Dementia Patient*. New York: Plenum Press, 1994.

Emery, Olga B., and Thomas E. Oxman. *Dementia: Presentations, Differential Diagnosis and Nosology*. Baltimore: Johns Hopkins University Press, 1994.

Erikson, E. H. *Identity and the Life Cycle*. New York: Norton, 1980.

Feil, Naomi. *The Validation Breakthrough: Simple Techniques for Communicating with People with "Alzheimer's Type Dementia."* Baltimore: Health Professions Press, 1993.

Gottfries, C. S., and S. Nakamura, eds. *Neurotransmitters and Dementia*. New York: Wien, 1990.

Gruetzner, Howard. *Alzheimer's: A Caregiver's Guide and Source Book*. New York: Wiley, 1992.

Guttman, Rosaline A. *Adult Care for Alzheimer's Patients: Impact on Family Caregivers*. New York: Garland, 1991.

Heston, Leonard L. *The Vanishing Mind: A Practical Guide to Alzheimer's Disease and Other Dementias*. New York: Freeman Press, 1991.

Huppert, Felicia A., Carol Brayne, and Daniel W. O'Conner, eds. *Dementia and Normal Aging*. New York: Cambridge University Press, 1994.

Levinson, D. *The Seasons of a Man's Life*. New York: Ballantine, 1978.

Light, E., G. Niederehe, and B. Lebowitz, eds. *Stress Effects on Family Caretakers of Alzheimer's Patients*. New York: Springer, 1994.

Lyman, Karen A. *Day in Day out with Alzheimer's: Stress in Caregiving Relationships*. Philadelphia: Temple University Press, 1993.

Mace, Nancy L. *The 36 Hour Day: A Family Guide to Caring for Persons with Alzheimer's Disease, Related Dementing Illnesses, and Memory Loss*. Baltimore: Johns Hopkins University Press, 1991.

McKay, Donald. *Sanctuary: A Care Center for Patients with Alzheimer's Disease*. Waterloo, Ontario: University of Waterloo Press, 1988.

Miller, Edgar, and Robin Morris. *The Psychology of Dementia*. New York: Wiley Press, 1993.

"New Alzheimer's Test Shows Promise." *Chicago Sun Times*, November 11, 1994.

Nitsch, Roger M., ed. *Alzheimer's Disease: Amyloid Precursor Proteins, Signal Transduction, and Neuronal Transplantation*. New York: New York Academy of Sciences Press, 1993.

Parks, R., R. Zec, and R. Wilson, eds. *Neuropsychology of Alzheimer's Disease and Other Dementias*. New York: Oxford University Press, 1993.

Peck, R. C. "Psychological Development in the Second Half of Life." In *Middle Age and Aging*, edited by B. L. Neugarlen. Chicago: University of Chicago Press, 1968.

Pollen, Daniel A. *Hannah's Heirs: The Quest for the Genetic Origins of Alzheimer's Disease*. New York: Oxford University Press, 1993.

Poon, L., ed. *Handbook for Clinical Memory Assessment of Older Adults*. Washington, D.C.: American Psychological Association, 1986.

Powell, Lenore S. *Alzheimer's Disease: A Guide for Families*. Reading, Mass.: Addison-Wesley Press, 1993.

Rau, Marie T. *Aging with Communication Challenges in Alzheimer's Disease*. San Diego: Singular Publishing Group, 1993.

Reeder, P., J. Fritze, and M. B. H. Youdin, eds. *Neuroprotection in Neurodegeneration*. New York: Wien, 1994.

Soukup, J. E. *Understanding and Living with Mental Illness in the Family*. Springfield, Ill.: Charles C. Thomas Publishers, 1995.

Storandt, Martha, and Gary R. VandenBos, eds. *Neuropsychological Assessment of Dementia and Depression in Older Adults: A Clinician's Guide*. Washington, D.C.: American Psychological Association, 1994.

Taira, Ellen D., ed. *The Mentally Impaired Elderly: Strategies and Interventions to Maintain Functions.* New York: Haworth Press, 1991.

Wright, Lore K. *Alzheimer's Disease and Marriage: An Intimate Account.* Newbury Park, N.J.: Sage Publications, 1993.

Zandi, Taker, and Richard J. Ham, eds. *New Directions in Understanding Dementia and Alzheimer's Disease.* New York: Plenum Press, 1990.

ASSESSMENT INSTRUMENTS

Beck, A. T. *Beck Hopelessness Scale.* San Antonio: The Psychological Corporation, Harcourt, Brace, Jovanovich, 1988.

Beck, A. T., and R. A. Steer. *The Beck Depression Inventory.* San Antonio: The Psychological Corporation, Harcourt, Brace, Jovanovich, 1987.

Dahlstrom, W. G., G. S. Welsh, and L. E. Dahlstrom. *Minnesota Multiphasic Personality Inventory.* Minneapolis: University of Minnesota Press, 1975.

Goodglass, H., and E. Kaplan. *The Assessment of Aphasia and Related Disorders.* Malvern, Pa.: Lea and Febiger, 1983.

Kaplan, E., D. Fein, R. Morris, and D. Delis. *Wechsler Adult Intelligence Scale—Revised—Neuropsychological Instrument.* San Antonio: The Psychological Corporation, Harcourt, Brace, Jovanovich, 1991.

Kaplan E., H. Goodglass, and S. Weintraub. *Boston Naming Test.* Malvern, Pa.: Lea and Febiger, 1983.

Wechsler, D. *Wechsler Adult Intelligence Scale—Revised.* San Antonio: The Psychological Corporation, Harcourt, Brace, Jovanovich, 1981.

» «

Index

ABOUT THE AUTHOR

JAMES E. SOUKUP is a licensed clinical psychologist in private practice. He specializes in the diagnosis, treatment, and management of Alzheimer's disease and other dementias. His other books include studies of attention-deficit disorder and the psychology of aging.

ISBN 0-275-95460-9

EAN

9 780275 954604

HARDCOVER BAR CODE